Raph BOOK ONE

Nature's Recipe
for
Peak Health

The Antidote for
Commercialized Medicine

MORNING: SPIRIT: WOLF, DRM

Nature's Recipe for Peak Health
By Morning: Spirit: Wolf- D.R.M.

www.raphaology.info
www.raphaology.tv
www.peakherbs.org
www.ifarmacy.com

Copyright © 2012 Morning: Spirit: Wolf- D.R.M.

All rights reserved. No part of this book may be reproduced or transmitted in any form or by any means, electronic or mechanical, including photocopying, recording, or by any information storage and retrieval system, without prior permission from the copyright owner, except for the inclusion of brief quotations in an article or review.

ISBN 978-0-9848457-0-5

First Edition
Library of Congress Cataloging-in Publication Data pending.

Cover design by
Barbara Goss Anderson, Two Hands2 Art & Design
Gwyn Snider, GKS Creative
gkscreative.com

Interior Design by
GKS Creative

Illustrations by
Molly Brown

Printed in the united states of America

Dedication

This work is dedicated to all earth's people and the life's purpose of Jonathan: Thunder: Wolf-D.R.M., who foresaw that new information and resources about health and healing were imperative for overcoming the degenerative dis-eases rampant today. Although Jonathan's work is completely independent from any other, it has been proven out in differing aspects by a number of brilliant people whose critical findings, like Jonathan's, are now becoming part of collective awareness and consciousness. May all the loving, creative, and life supporting elements of the universe be manifest in the awareness of humanity and implemented with joy.

Appreciation

With profound appreciation for Molly Brown, whose young talent, insight, and feel for human bio-dynamics are extraordinary, as are her intuitively rendered illustrations in this book. Molly, you are the embodiment of altruism. For your passionate donation of time, energy and considerable skills that lend matchless quality to the imagery of this book, my admiration and heartfelt thankfulness are yours.

Thanks

For the generous time, talents, patience, skills and efforts of the caliber of extraordinary people who have supported the production of this work, infinite thanks, recognition, and genuine gratefulness are offered: Khohala, for holding me tenderly within your hands, gently sharing the collective purpose; Antoinette, for your friendship, encouragement, praise and constructive assessment alike; Sion, for your listening ear; Natalie, for your astute input; Bryn, for your love in the face of adversity, to name but a few to whom thanks are abundantly deserved.

Gratuity

Jonathan and Morning have been the grateful recipients of answers offered by wizened giants, both sung and unsung, that have gone before us. If there is good that results from the efforts contained herein, we, like Isaac Newton, can only claim to have stood on the shoulders of giants to get a better view.

Table of Contents

Foreword

I have walked the path that I am directing you to. Dis-ease is a silent protest of the body, pleading for your attention. I was diagnosed with fibromyalgia, limiting my ability to work as a full time anesthesiologist or to exert myself in my day-to-day activities. I wanted to deal with the dis-ease and get my vitality back rather than just treating the various symptoms, and I succeeded. I chose the privilege of healing it with naturaceuticals of Raphaology: herbs, food and stress reduction. It was a nontoxic journey to healing, and release, not toward just suppression of symptoms. Become nurturing toward your body and give it the best dependable support, then it gives back to you. Gauge your journey with the depth of your breathing, the relaxing rhythm of your heart and the glow in your eyes, which reflect your physical, emotional and spiritual progress respectively.

Our health is a finely tuned balance of our physical, emotional, psychological and spiritual strengths. These strengths in variable proportions determine our individual persona and our own acuity in regulating and responding to our environment. Our health is affected by a permutation and combination of various assaults caused on us by our environment and our ability to defend ourselves.

Our body is a composition of well-regulated systems, kept properly working by specific glandular hormones and enzymes that play a key role in preserving our health. To empower our body to serve us optimally, we have to be judicious gatekeepers of what goes into our body, its source, its nutritional strength, its potency and its effects, both beneficial and detrimental.

We have started to lean heavily on statistical analysis of studies done on pockets of society, which may or may not apply to the whole. Do we ever question ourselves — " Am I interested in just treating, and/or suppressing my symptoms or do I want to use tools to empower my body's innate ability to heal itself"? Our lifestyles have contributed to the increased incidence of diabetes, hypertension, and heart disease. The absence of nutritive elements in food and the presence of added multiple stresses further deplete our body of vital energy.

There is a shift, and we have entered an era where the art and science of self-healing is being sought for. There is fresh awareness of different modalities that one can intertwine to help us on this journey. Dr. Morning: Spirit: Wolf shares her longstanding experience of three decades and her wide scope of knowledge compiled over the years to provide us with guidelines, explanations and tools for this exciting journey we all should be encouraged to take.

PARAMJIT BHALLA M.D.

Author's Note

Health, which involves our physical, emotional, and spiritual selves, is our birthright, but it's also a choice. We can opt to lead healthy, regenerative lives or we can practice habits that deplete us. And with more than 50 percent of us overweight, with heart dis-ease and Type II diabetes rampant, there is little doubt that many of us are making the convenient choice, leading to degeneration, rather than the wise choice, leading to regeneration. There is no doubt that our eating habits, which determine our health index, are driven by advertising, persuasion, and expediency; that our priorities are skewed in ways that make our lives too stressful; that we have lost touch with the importance of self-nurture.

And then there is more advertising. Advertising telling us that when we overeat degenerative foods, there are pills that can cure everything from high blood pressure to acid reflux; that can manage everything from high cholesterol to Type II diabetes. And not knowing what else to do, we buy into it, creating a multi-billion dollar a year drug industry where a few small changes in what we consume and how we consume it could make a huge difference—could truly regenerate and maintain our health and well-being.

If you have opened this book, you are looking for solutions. And you will find them. Adopting them is another story. Do you have the desire to maximize your health? And in so doing, to maximize your overall well-being? Do you have the discipline to read through and learn about your body, its integration with your spirit, and what it takes to truly nourish all three? Are you ready to open your mind to the opportunity for genuine health, regardless of where you are now?

Raphaology is not a diet. It is an encompassing lifestyle

that teaches you all you need to know to optimize your health. And it requires that you take accountability for doing so. This is serious fun.

We all know when we don't feel well, but what did it take to get you there? When we feel sick, the symptoms of headache, stomach pain, or tiredness are our body's way of telling us that our toxic choices in food, drinks, stress, work, etc. have caught up with us. The body needs to dispose of the toxins we've accumulated, and each symptom is the body demonstrating the process of toxins or pathogens leaving. In the case of simply detoxifying the energy drink you just drank, your sickness will be over in an hour, but if your sickness is a build-up of all the energy drinks, burgers, pastries, apples, oatmeal, peanut butter, chicken, white bread, and celery you composted in your colon over the past years, feeding hosts of parasites, then you are going to need help.

What you are going to learn is how to attain, maintain, and prolong the health and function of every part of your body. It's not just about keeping you operational, but maximizing your capacity, slowing your aging process, and peaking your performance.

The ancient wisdoms and revitalized insights in this book are offered as a means to educate and inform with the highest intent for each of us to access and utilize our innate ability for healing and experiencing joy.

The context of information contained herein has not been evaluated or approved by the FDA and is not intended to diagnose, treat, or control disease. Rather, it is intended to reveal the time-tested methods, resources, and factors that can assist each individual in choosing accountability and exercising their ability for self-healing. In the event that individuals use any of the information in this book for healing purposes, the author and publisher assume no responsibility for your individual actions, but heartily support your right to self-heal.

Once each of us uncovers our inner doctor and awakens to the healing power that is innately part of our inherent, genetic, and spiritual heritage, a consciousness raising occurs, putting us in touch with higher powers that transcend the bounds of science and math, connecting us to the unseen, unheard worlds where only ease exists. It is the goal of this work to assist individuals in achieving freedom from dis-ease and any other imposed bounds.

> *"A healthy body is a guest chamber for the soul:*
> *a sick body a prison."*
> FRANCIS BACON SR.

Classic Hippocratic Oath of Medicine
(TRANSLATION FROM ORIGINAL GREEK)

I swear by Apollo Physician and Asclepius and Hygieia and Panaceia and all the gods and goddesses, making them my witness, that I will fulfill according to my ability and judgment this oath and this covenant:

To hold him who has taught me this art as equal to my parents and to live my life in partnership with him, and if he is in need of money to give him a share of mine, and to regard his offspring as equal to my brothers in male lineage and to teach them this art—if they desire to learn it—without fee and covenant; to give a share of precepts and oral instruction and all other learning to my sons and to the sons of him who has instructed me and to pupils who have signed the covenant and have taken an oath according to the medical law, but no one else.

I will apply nutritional measures for the benefit of the sick according to my ability and judgment; I will keep them from harm and injustice.

I will neither give deadly drug to anybody who asked for it, nor will I make suggestion to this effect. Similarly I will not give to a woman an abortive remedy. In purity and holiness I will guard my life and art.

I will not use the knife, not even on sufferers from stone, but will withdraw in favor of such men as are engaged in this work.

I will remember that there is art as well as science to medicine and using warmth, sympathy, and understanding may outweigh the surgeon's knife or the chemist's drug.

I will strive to prevent disease whenever I can, for prevention is preferable to cure.

Whatever houses I may visit, I will come in benefit of the

sick, remaining free of all intentional injustice, of all mischief and in particular of sexual relations with both female and male persons, be they free or slaves.

I will remember that I do not treat a fever chart, a cancerous growth, but a sick human being, whose illness may affect the person's family and economic stability.

What I may see or hear in the course of the treatment or even outside of the treatment in regard to the life of men, which on no account one must spread abroad, I will keep to myself, holding such things shameful to be spoken about.

If I fulfill this oath and do not violate it, may it be granted to me to enjoy life and art, being honored with fame among all men for all time to come; if I transgress it and swear falsely, may the opposite of all this be my lot.

Jumping In

I am alive, powerful, and healthy, but I wasn't always that way.

Imagine that you are seventeen years old and you wake up to find most of the hair that was on your head is now on the pillow. And you didn't have chemotherapy. Imagine being frightened of food because an unknown quantity might make your lungs collapse, your heart stop, and your eyes swell shut. Imagine being afraid that the arthritis on your right side might cripple the rest of you too. Then, in college, having one of your chronic sinus infections break through the sinus cavities and go into your already pounding brain, rendering you a temporary vegetable. Imagine enduring years of antibiotics, antihistamines, diuretics, steroids, anti-inflammatories, pain meds and struggling with the backlash of side effects. Doctor after doctor, test after test, still in kidney failure, and it's not getting any better. That was my life. I was worn out. Then the prognosis got worse: my doctor told me I was going to die. Blood clots and a liver tumor were to be my murderers. Not exactly something a free spirited girl looks forward to.

I was angry. I was scared. Hadn't I done everything the doctors told me to do? I wasn't ready to be dead. I was fed up with the doctors attitudes and platitudes assuring me they had done everything short of the cure. I may have been defenseless but I wasn't a wimp.

So all things considered, I fired my doctor. Then he conveyed the greatest gift. He looked me in the eye and said "You can't fire me, you don't know what you're doing. You'll be taking your life into your own hands." The irony of that statement blew me away. I knew then and there that if I truly wanted to live I was going to have to take charge of my life. I didn't know what I was going to do, or how I was going to do it, but I wasn't going down without a fight. So I strapped on an iron will and set off for parts unknown.

Trying every out-of-the-box, electro-magnetic, Oriental fuzzy gray bark, liquid diet, bitter berry remedy I could find, my health made slight improvements. I was headed in the right direction. But when Jonathan: Thunder: Wolf hit my radar I truly became a hopeful skeptic. I had heard he was a healer of the un-heal-able, but could it be applicable to me? I had to give it a try. I had nothing to lose.

His strategy was straightforward, his method was impressive, his prognosis was positive, and everything was natural. Upon giving Jonathan's food and herb recommendations a fully fledged try, I began to improve and feel stronger, a little more every day. This was good. And it kept getting better.

I became a healing machine. I took sarsaparilla for my kidneys, and ate lots of papaya. Hawthorn leaf was for my liver, and red beets and noni shrunk the tumor. I had so many B-Complex vitamins that my sweat began to smell like it. Vitamin E and alfalfa took care of the blood clots, while iron from nettles replenished my energy. I took marjoram for my sinuses, plus cayenne and chamomile for the infections. American ginseng kept the oxygen flowing to the cells and eliminated lung fluids along with yerba santa. Thyme tea for my digestion became a best friend and I tried mango and goat cheese for the first time in my life. Horsetail silica kept the excess fluids at bay and juniper berry fought off the arthritis. And while I had been trained to be afraid of fats, extra virgin olive oil and avocados were daily champions that proved to help my body metabolize the minerals I needed to rebuild.

Less than 2 years later I had:
- Kidneys that were fully functional
- No blood clots or tumors
- Allergies and arthritis gone
- Sinus infections eliminated

- More energy than I knew what to do with

And for the first time in my life I was clear headed, had a wonderful sense of well being, and I felt sexier. Maybe that last one had something to do with why I married Jonathan, my hero.

Raphaology is still my daily medicine. After nearly 30 years of living it, practicing and teaching its principles, assisting others find their health with it, Raphaology still excites me. It works.

And now I am sharing what Jonathan and I learned. Welcome to the world of healing. Welcome to Raphaology.

Where To Begin

*"A man too busy to take care of his health
is like a mechanic too busy to take care of his tools."*
SPANISH PROVERB

NOT EVERYONE is faced with having to make a save-your-life or accept death decision. But if you are, or know someone who is, you will find answers here. If you are already healthy, or simply curious about a superior, healthier lifestyle, the answers for that are here too. Get ready to be excited.

Your body is an automatic, self-healing organism designed for perpetual health. Yet, commercial medicine disregards and obscures this universal principle. Modern medicine has its merits; it *is* designed to help you in an emergency. It is *not* designed to keep you well. Raphaology is. As modern medicine has developed we have acceded our innate healing ability to scientific medicine, especially in crisis. Moreover, we have acceded our responsibility to maintain our health, instead counting on medications and the medical community to compensate for the poor habits we have developed. It's time to take back control. Raphaology is here to provide you with the tools to do so, to revest you with the power that has always been yours.

Dis-ease is not inevitable. When know-how, attention, lubrication, and maintenance is not applied, even the best machinery will break down. Your body is an organic mechanism requiring awareness, care, nourishment, and maintenance using elements compatible with its natural origins. Raphaology provides the information and the tools so you need never break down, get ill, or be threatened with a deadly dis-ease.

Regardless of your current state of health, you will find Raphaology advantageous. If you're well now, adopting the Raphaology lifestyle will keep you there; if you're sick, following the contained information will enable you to get well. No matter if you're in your twenties or your eighties, Raphaology is a comprehensive health style that will inform, empower, and provide resources for every aspect of your body, mind, and infinite life source.

Modern medicine treats us as victims of illness. We are not. All dis-eases can be prevented and cured. Limiting our belief in the body's ability to heal itself limits our healing capacity, rendering us emotionally and functionally impotent to steer our health on even the most basic levels.

The question is, do you want to do something about it? Do you want an antidote for the inferior information, the invasive measures, and the overwhelming sense of impotence that are sullying your health?

Healing takes place when the mind knows the answers, the body accepts the correct response, especially in emergencies so that panic doesn't take over, and the infinite life source of the soul motivates action for health with positive feelings that support it. Your body is designed to tell your mind what it needs. Raphaology will teach you how to listen, how to respond, and provide the tools to do so.

Raphaology provides you with the natural antidote for both the information and the invasive measures that have compromised your intelligence and your health. Reading this book will make you ready to re-evaluate the current health care system, and after seeing how it can lead to further dis-ease, will reveal that your innate healing system possesses every ability to heal from any dis-ease.

Raphaology is a revolutionary healing art that encompasses ancient aspects of indigenous healing methods, which hold the keys for transforming our every cell, our very DNA, allowing new energetic patterns of information, focus, and purpose to unlock abilities we have only dreamed of. Raphaology is nature's true medicine, the antidote for commercial medicine.

> **Raphaology** is a revolutionary art that encompasses ancient aspects of indigenous healing methods.

Raphaology uses specific plants that possess the medicinal properties that enable the repairing and regenerating functions of the human body to revitalize health. The world at large perceives medicine vastly differently from the western world. Many countries use herbs as their first line of defense and drugs as a last resort. As a matter of fact, international law defines medicine as *"healing practices, without surgery or invasion, using medicines that heal or cure a disease process."*

In commercial medicine it is symptoms, not causes, that are the focus of practice, using invasive measures to remove blood or tissue to laboratories, or injecting caustic dyes or radiations to determine appropriate pharmaceutical treatment, which produces inhibiting, blocking, and masking consequences and harmful side-effects, while leaving the root cause to further degenerate. Instead, Raphaology involves hands-on access of nerve path connections to internal organs. This method provides clear information, without invasive measures, for determining the root cause of symptoms. Then herbal properties are implemented to repair the causative problem and eliminate its symptoms.

The Raphaology approach

> You, indeed, **are** what you eat.

qualifies each dis-ease and its resulting symptom as a digestive system malfunction. When a food substance has not been digested or eliminated, its stored components putrefy, producing toxic off gasses along with the host environment for antibody growth. Stored nutrients become depleted by fending off toxins and pathogens, which become prolific and then are transported in blood fluids throughout the body and become dis-easement where they lodge. If those poisons or harmful microorganisms stay in the lungs, modern medicine may call this symptom asthma; in the joints its symptom is termed arthritis; in the pancreas it's labeled as pancreatitis or diabetes; in the sinuses it's called allergies or sinusitis; in the bones it may be named osteoporosis; and so on. Every symptom of ill health begins as malnutrition, a deficiency of nutrients that sustain healthy function.

Within these pages you will learn how your body functions, how it dysfunctions, how to recognize a problem, and how to restore health. You will be taught healing herbs and foods, how to prevent dis-ease, and how to practice the cure. You will learn that dis-ease is simply a loss of minerals and what to do, eat, drink, and think to get them back. You will gain knowledge to transform your normal life into glowing health and vital living.

> Every symptom of ill health **begins** as malnutrition, a deficiency of nutrients that sustain **healthy** function.

What follows are out-of-the-box, extraordinary, un-conventional views and applications for real healing. Prepare to have your belief systems challenged and your knowledge of health de-term-inated.

Do We Need a Guide?

"A man who wants something will find a way;
a man who doesn't will find an excuse."
STEPHEN DOLLEY JR.

LET'S FACE IT. None of us come with an instruction manual, or if we did it has long since been lost. We are figuring it out as we go, doing the best we can with the information at hand. But with our busy lives — and the barrage of conflicting information, where do we find the time and expertise to distill what is best, what will truly maximize our health?

We seem to have awakened to the dangers of preservatives, additives, and artificial colors and there is a heightened awareness of the benefits of fruits and vegetables and of organic foods. But what we seem to have lost is our innate knowledge of the healing properties of plants and foods. And in a society that is ready to turn away from artificial foods and back to purer nutrition, the time is right for education about something our ancestors understood. Certain plants actually heal.

> What we seem to have lost is our innate **knowledge** of the healing properties of plants and **foods.**

Raphaology is the guide that encompasses healing with knowledge of medicinal plants with their applications brought forward from ancient practices in hundreds of nations over thousands of years. The teachings of Raphaology have a long history, but also include recent exhaustive studies and testing, conducted to apply its principles to current planetary conditions and human lifestyles. In short, Raphaology encompasses the best of traditional healing, complementary to today's conditions for the most peak results.

To start with practical ways to guide you through this exciting and life-enhancing process, let's look a little deeper than the surface. Most of us are intuitive beings, but in our modern world the intuitive powers have been suppressed. Being constantly inundated and persuaded by mass media and marketing programs it is possible the intuitive, energetic part of us is forgotten and no longer communicates with the physical except through emotions, which the brain has been taught to disregard as inferior. You, the intuitive energetic being with the real power, may be ignored, but you are not forgotten. You are still in there somewhere. The energetic part of you is the real you, and it is emerging into a new paradigm.

> The intuitive, **energetic** part of us is forgotten and no longer communicates with the physical except through **emotions**, which the brain has been taught to disregard.

You, the energetic, infinite life source of the soul that gives life to the physical body, are using that body as your vehicle to participate in the material world. You are not your body. You are also not your brain. The brain can only know what it takes in through its five senses: what it sees, hears, tastes, smells, and touches. It makes no distinction of right or wrong, good or bad. It just takes in the differing information as facts. While the brain knows what it has been taught, your heart, the physical part of you that connects to your infinite life source, knows and recognizes the truth.

Your heart converts and makes all the electricity for your body, those energy patterns of electrical currents known as e-motions (energy motions) that pass along information to and from every cell of you, not just the brain cells. Unlike the brain which passes along external information *to* the inside of you, your heart *knows* all the information on the inside of you. Electronically the heart is in constant communication with each body cell and always chooses to feel what is right for you—those positive, healthy, happy, joyful, inspirational e-motions—and even gets excited about it. It's time you started to use your brain for what it was designed for—internalizing sensory information about the outside world—and begin to go inside, in to it, to your intuition by listening to your heart, so that you can know the truth about *you*, including innate healing know-how. The intuitive energetic you is the true you, the endless, ageless, abundant, creative you, whereas your brain's experiences have been conditioned by the situations and occurrences of things outside of you.

A New Beginning

*" A bright future for man is spending less time
proving that he can outwit nature and more time
tasting her sweetness and respecting her seniority."*

E.B. WHITE 1945

IT'S A GOOD TIME to be alive! No matter where you live. Those of us who live in the modern world get to experience on a daily basis the wonders of technology, science, and medicine — but instead of suffering the consequences of those modern wonders, let's turn it around. Instead of depending more on computers and technology that harm us with radiation, let's rely on our own life experience know-how. Instead of depending on telephones, e-mail, and texting to keep us in touch, let's share a touch or laugh in the flesh. Instead of relying on agri-business to feed us their genetically modified, synthetically amended, irradiated, and nutrient-less foods, let's grow and know our own nourishment. Let's stop depending on marketing companies to dictate trends on "what's in" to buy, eat, drive, invest, think, and wear, and start forming our own perceptions based on what feels right. Let's stop depending on medical doctors and pharmaceuticals to diagnose and treat our symptoms, and start taking accountability for our own health. Let's stop abandoning our own truth, health, and abilities to large multinational chemical corporations, social and financial systems, and technological mechanisms and become the joyous, self-sustaining race of beings we were created to be.

We can become independent rather than dependent. Let's not cede our independence, the hallmark of humanity, to convenience. It's time to reclaim our independence and self empowerment. We, as a race of humanity have reached our critical threshold, with ignorance, poverty, disease, and fear at an all time high. It's time for the pendulum to swing in the opposite direction. It's time to be independent of ignorance, manipulation, fear and disease. It's time for abundance, passion, health, freedom, and creativity. It's time to have everything we want, becoming once again savvy as to what those wants could be. Our health is our wealth. Our basis for a transformation in healing comes with knowledge.

Knowledge is power. Raphaology precepts are power-packed with practical, useful, and readily applicable tools that are intended to wake us up from the mindless fog we have been lulled into. Within Raphaology can be found the relevant, practical information, motivation, and means for reclaiming health, passion, and independence from modern marketing, and commercialized pressure, persuasion, and manipulation. With re-empowerment and healing tools we have the perfect combination for vital and dynamic living, thinking, feeling, perceiving, choosing, acting, relating, and creating, all without fear.

What is Raphaology and Where Did It Come From?

"The doctor of the future will give no medicine,
but will interest his patients in the care of human frame,
and in the cause and prevention of disease."

THOMAS E. EDISON

RAPHAOLOGY, pronounced *raw-fah-all-oh-gee*, has its roots in the study and practice of light and all its healing aspects from ancient and modern sources. The combined applications of past and present natural healing arts offers the return of light as the medium for integrating the physical, emotional, mental, and infinite life source (spirit) of every individual, facilitating the most peak healing.

Indigenous teachers and practitioners of ancient healing have held sacred the knowledge of the repairing aspects of herb and food properties for absolute health by repairing, restoring, boosting, and maintaining every body function. Raphaology offers this revitalized information and methods for self-healing, applications and tools that facilitate repairing of the cellular body, restoration of degenerated systems, balancing of hormones, and unifying us with light—our life source. Today, Raphaology wisdoms provide real and simple solutions for creating a healthy, peaceful, and enhanced atmosphere for joyful living from the often unhealthy, confusing, and limiting world that we currently share.

Raphaology is a combination of four component parts:

1. Herbs - plants that provide medicinal properties
2. Foods - fuel with specific enzymes and nutrients
3. ID Therapy - an interactive system for determining internal conditions
4. Color Therapy - light spectrum frequencies that govern hormones

These simple and natural components work together to determine and provide any missing nutrients, elements, or co-factors of the body, which begins the healing process. After the missing component has been replaced, it is not unusual for the negative symptoms of the body to disappear, whether it be physical symptoms, hormonal imbalances, or psychological problems. Then renewed energy, clear thought, emotional stability, total immunity, and increased longevity and vitality can be restored.

Having practical tools for integrating your mind, body, emotions, and infinite life source with the rest of the living universe allows you to feel whole; complete within your self and secure with being and acting on your part of the whole.

Founded by Jonathan: Thunder: Wolf, as a means of saving his life, Raphaology began as one man's search for answers. I later joined in the search as I began a journey to save my own life. Basing the name of Raphaology in ancient frequencies found in languages used by indigenous peoples both long ago and today, it is derived from a combination of two ancient words:

RA, the knowledge of progressing a planet to its peak frequency as a sun,
and
PHA, the knowledge of bringing peak frequency light to all matter.

RAPHAOLOGY *Nature's Antidote for Commercialized Medicine*

Raphaology is a new study of lost powers and how their applications benefit the practical world today. These two simple premises contain universal knowledge that provide the basis for healing on every level.

You may find that the use of Raphaology information, herbs, and foods, which hold high concentrations of light, and applying the understanding that light is energy and energy is knowledge, will give your body, mind, and emotions new light, energy and knowledge and restore understanding, memories, and abilities to your life.

Changing your health starts with your desire and intention to change for the better. If you hadn't already made the decision for positive change you wouldn't be reading this book. Now you can start to act on your own behalf, acquiring new information on how to change your life for the better, how to heal yourself, and what tools to use for doing so. Your body already knows what it should be doing. It's time for your brain to catch up.

> Changing your **health** starts with your desire and intention to **change** for the better.

How It Works

"Health is a state of complete physical, mental, and social well-being, and not merely the absence of disease or infirmity."

WORLD HEALTH ORGANIZATION 1948

OUR HUMAN BODIES are organic, natural, health-seeking, automatically repairing mechanisms that will always choose ease over dis-ease, therefore capable of replacing stored inferior materials with superior elements. Observing our skin heal before our very eyes is the visual proof. Every time we see our skin heal from a cut, bruise, burn, rash, or infection it is showing us that we have the ability to repair, on the inside as well as out. When we supply the body with energy-infused, healthful, life-enhancing, superior elements, our bodies can do what they are created to do: heal and sustain vital energy.

> Our human **bodies** are organic, natural, health-seeking, automatically **repairing** mechanisms that will always choose ease over dis-ease.

We are composed of cells of all types: tissue, bone, muscle, organ, hair, etc. More than that, we are electromagnetic in nature. Overall the body is a living, energetic miracle! We each started out as a single cell that divided into two, then four, and so on. Did you ever stop to wonder how all those cells knew to separate into the individual forms and features of our body? Or that each individual body cell contains enough information to totally reproduce you in your entirety?

Every cell is loaded with information, intelligence, and living energy. Each and every cell knows what it is doing, and how to do it. If the body's cells know how to create themselves, they certainly know how to heal themselves. Just as your external skin tissues prove to you on a daily basis that they repair damage before your very eyes, this same healing process takes place in our internal organs, bones, nerves and systems. Our bodies know enough to be immune to every disease, and they have the ability to heal from every dis-ease. All we have to do is supply the tools to facilitate healing.

LIGHT & HORMONES

That tool is light. We are light beings. Yes, we need air and water as well, but our bodies depend on light as the material from which to make hormones. Hormones are those vaporous substances that literally fuel every single function of our bodies. Each hormone gland makes its hormones from light. There are seven main hormone producing glands inside our bodies, and there are seven colors in the visible light spectrum. No coincidence there. Each of the seven glands uses one of the seven colors, or frequencies, from which to manufacture its hormones.

> Our **bodies** depend on light as the material from which to make **hormones**.

- **Pituitary gland**, located in the brain, uses gold light
- **Pineal gland**, also in the brain behind the eyes, uses yellow light

- **Thyroid**, in the base of the throat, uses green light
- **Mammary glands**, located in the nipples, use blue light
- **Kidneys and Adrenals**, at both sides of the back at the waist, use violet light
- **Pancreas**, on the left just above the navel, uses orange light
- **Testes and Ovaries**, located at the groin pelvic area; men's on the outside and women's on the inside, use the red spectrum of light

Hormones are the key to every organ function. Every organ depends on hormones as its fuel. Hormones make it possible to: digest food, circulate the nutrients and the oxygen, eliminate waste and toxins, think our thoughts, understand our experiences, make our decisions, feel and share our emotions, act on our intelligence, and create and manifest our intentions. Without light and the subsequent hormones it becomes, we experience some degree of dis-ease in every organ and system. With light we experience health, vitality, passion, and the ability to truly live.

> Every **organ** depends on hormones as its **fuel**.

Hormones enhance our abilities and absence of hormones produces our disabilities. When we have enough light we have positive emotions, proper organ function, balanced systems, and live closer to our true nature. When we have light deficiency we experience the opposite and concurrent negative aspects of the mind, body, emotions, and spirit, causing us to accept and live with artificial emotions, health, and realities.

> Hormones **enhance** our abilities and absence of **hormones** produces our disabilities.

In other words, using our abilities as light beings brings us knowledge, health, joy, balance, freedom, creativity, and peace. All of this feels good to us because that is who, what, how, why, when, and where we really are: pure light energy with the ability to take on any form, function, or purpose we choose.

Hormones are responsible for the tiny little light bodies known as—"somatids"—that are the life source for each individual cell in your body. Just as your physical body as a whole is enlivened by your soul body, the individual cells of your body each have a soul body. These Somatids comprise the energy that sustains the power source of each cell. They are so tiny that they can only be viewed under live, dark field microscopic magnification. Yet they produce profound energy sources. Under these conditions it can be observed that Somatids travel through our blood fluids, lymphatic fluids, and cellular fluids and *are* literally that spark of life, twinkle in the eye, or vital life force presence that is purely energetic in nature. This accounts for why people who have true vitality have balanced hormones, and also why these individuals have that certain quality you can't quite put your finger on. You just feel that they have something special.

Too much foo-foo stuff for you? Hang in there, it gets more practical.

The Physics of Light

*"Ultimately, in physics, you're hoping to convince Nature.
And I've found Nature to be pretty reasonable."*
FRANK WILCZEK 1978

A RUSSIAN MECHANICAL ENGINEER with Ph.D.'s in physics and geology first heard about Raphaology from his wife, who was my patient. He had studied light in its various forms, and had an educated understanding of its properties, so he was skeptical about her explanation that different colors in the light spectrum could be used by the body for healing. He was, however, curious to meet someone with no formal education on the subject who had educated her about this.

At first contact he was dubious, but with his considerable knowledge he could ask intelligent and compelling questions. Since I love a challenge, and offered considerable experience in the practicalities of light and its healing abilities, we were mutually impressed and hit it off immediately. We had many late night discussions, which included some interchanges that got fairly deep and provocative. What follows emanates from some of our discussion material.

It is known in physics that the rays of light from the sun contain all frequencies, seen and unseen, which includes all minerals, vitamins, and nutrients. These nutrients, as rays of sunlight, are pure white light energy in the form of frequency bands that vibrate at different speeds and spans; in sound technology they are called wave length and amplitude. Separating out the different vibratory rates, or wave frequencies, produces visual color spectrum differences, which if recombined will result in their perfect balance: white light.

PRISMATIC FLUID & AURIC FIELDS

The human body is composed of 80 percent water — every cell floats in cellular fluid. Each drop of cellular fluid, like a raindrop, is prismatic in nature. In the same way that white light from sunshine penetrates a raindrop and is separated into a rainbow of colors, each drop of fluid in the human body receives light and separates it into the spectrum of colors that are used to manufacture hormones. So not only is water the medium of exchange and delivery of nutrients and waste, water provides the element for the absorption, separation, usage, and expression of light: the human aura field.

Each and every cell in our bodies floats in cellular water composed of liquid light crystals. Dr. Masaru Emoto showed the world that there are energies in water that can rearrange themselves into perfect geometric form by absorbing the frequencies of words like *love* and *appreciation*. The intelligent and highly whetable medium of both earth and human fluids can crystallize dirty water into glowing jewels of joy when offered higher frequencies than what they currently hold.

When we renew the body fluids by drinking good quality water, such as mountain spring or

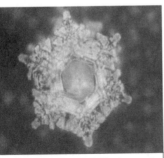

Masaru Emoto's dark field microscopic photography depicting the structure of cellular fluid after responding to the affixation of a simple "thank you" onto a jar of polluted water, transforming chaotic fluid into beautiful geometric, pH form.

glacier water, it charges body cells with pulsating life force and the cellular fluid with the perfect medium for expelling carbon dioxide, toxic off-gasses, and cellular waste, while delivering fresh oxygen, enlivened nutrients, and a renewal of function and activity. We can make our own quality water by affixing high frequency words to the water's container.

For every cell type there is a particular structure to the fluid around it that determines how the cell responds. The ripple effect of both pH-balanced and light-charged cellular fluid extends to every part of your body—from signaling immune response to marshalling forces for defense, or providing the perfect medium to deliver life force factors to each cell and carrying away cellular waste.

Each cell requires an exchange of one specific color of light energy as its power source. Just as a car needs a battery, every particle of human anatomy needs the sun as its energy source. Plants use photosynthesis, the process of converting sunlight into chlorophyll. Human biochemical gland cells convert bio-available light into hormones, enzymes, vitamins, minerals, and other life force factors, which fuel every one of the many functions of each cell group.

Every ounce of quality liquid light-mineral rich, pH-balanced, living water that we provide our bodies improves, extends, enriches, and empowers each aspect of us to function at higher and higher levels of living. Light equals life.

The cycle of light in the human body

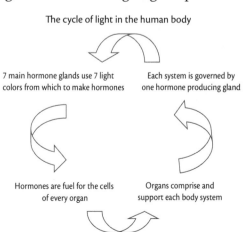

7 main hormone glands use 7 light colors from which to make hormones

Each system is governed by one hormone producing gland

Hormones are fuel for the cells of every organ

Organs comprise and support each body system

We have two main ways of receiving light: directly from the sun, and indirectly through the plants we ingest that contain sunlight. Light waves, or spectrum frequencies, from the sun, including ultra-violet rays, provide energy for plants to photosynthesize the products necessary for growth in the same way that light waves provide energy for humans to produce hormones and manufacture biological combustion and metabolism.

> We have two main ways of **receiving** light: directly from the sun, and indirectly through the plants we ingest that contain **sunlight**.

Because we live on light rather than matter, and all light is energy, it is light in waves of vibrating energy that become particles of matter within a magnetic field. Thus light is energy information as matter. For this reason the terms energy, light and information may be used synonymously and interchangeably.

MINERAL LIGHT

Each vibration, frequency, and color of light contains every specific vitamin, mineral and nutrient that fuels the human body. Of all the nutrients that are contained in light we humans, and every other living thing, need minerals as the bottom line in order to maintain life and the quality of performance.

All other nutrients—enzymes, sugars, vitamins, proteins, and fats—are conduits that get us to the final destination: minerals. Minerals are literally crystallized light. Every dis-ease is a mineral deficiency and, thus, a light deficiency.

> **Minerals** are the most vitally important element for **sustaining** our lives and maintaining quality of **life**.

All minerals absorb and give off light waves. These light waves, in the form of particles of minerals, work to keep us in peak health by providing all the supportive components to

Relationship of Visible Light to Other Wave Frequencies

Demonstrating the scope of rays and waves in scale to visible colors
that correspond with magnetic field, or point of gravity.

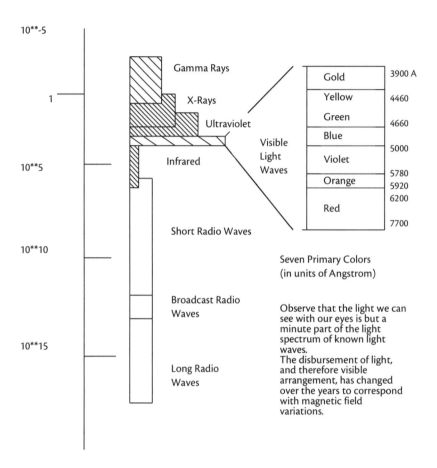

Seven Primary Colors
(in units of Angstrom)

Observe that the light we can
see with our eyes is but a
minute part of the light
spectrum of known light
waves.
The disbursement of light,
and therefore visible
arrangement, has changed
over the years to correspond
with magnetic field
variations.

The electromagnetic spectrum showing the relationship between visible "light" and other wavelengths of radiant information. Adapted from *Crystallography and Crystal Chemistry*, F. Donald Bloss.

maintain life. Any degree of mineral — or light — deficiency will produce dis-function, de-formities, and dis-ease. Minerals work at the cellular level and have the ability to neutralize acidity, toxicity, and anaerobic (without oxygen) activity, and restore all function and action to every cell. Since we are made of cells, their individual fate becomes our own.

> Every **dis-ease** is a mineral deficiency and, thus, a light deficiency.

If we have inadvertently depleted our minerals with chronic stress and the use of synthetic food, supplements, and drugs, including food drugs such as caffeine, fluoridated water, synthetic multi-vitamin/minerals supplements, and refined sugar and salt, we have effectively absorbed distorted light wavelengths. Distorted light is distorted minerals, which causes cell mutation and cell death, causing all dis-ease processes including cancerous growth and heart failure. On the other hand, specific organic plant-based minerals absorb full-spectrum light wavelengths that facilitate the body's electrical system (e.g. the heart) and enhance cellular functions. Organic minerals remove distortion and cell mutation, replacing it with pure energy in the form of electron activity.

Concentration of the sun's energy is improved when food rich in electrons (enzymes) are consumed. Electrons have a negative charge and orbit around nuclei that have a positive charge. Elec-

> The **electrons** of cells serve as the resonance system for the sun's **energy**.

trons in motion produce an electrical charge, which in turn creates a magnetic field. When they both interact an electrical circuit is produced. It is this current of energy that keeps the neurons sparking, the heart ticking, and the blood circulating; in other words, all systems firing.

7

Does This Relate?

"Those who dance are considered insane
by those who cannot hear the music."
GEORGE CARLIN

SINCE OUR RUSSIAN PHYSICIST was suffering from stomach ulcers that modern medicine had not been able to benefit, we tackled other areas of the body that are favored directly by sun's light frequencies. I explained that his stressed thinking was excessively over-stimulated, which in turn over-stimulated the stomach and exhausted the pancreas, which governs the stomach. He didn't get it until I explained that thoughts cause brain chemistry to effect all other body chemistry. Stressed thoughts create stressed digestion, which as interpreted by the pineal gland in the brain, produces excess or imbalanced stomach acid.

The pineal gland, located behind the eyes, is the body's light meter and its bio-rhythm regulator. The pituitary gland, located in the same area, is also stimulated and governed by light. These two glands monitor and supervise the entire endocrine system, defense system, life cycles and rhythms, and aging factors. Health of these glands and the proper balance of light waves, or frequencies, are, among other things, major factors in the prevention of many of today's light deficient diseases such as cancers, chronic fatigue, ulcers, bowel problems, and so forth.

Because his work was indoors, as an "inside" man Mr. Physicist was suffering from "mal-illumination"; dis-ease from artificial light. With his condition compounded by pollution, stress, and food toxins it caused him to suffer from chronic "mal-illumination," which, like malnutrition, creates major imbalances in the ability to produce balanced hormones and function as a healthy human being.

Dr. Fritz Hollowich conducted a 1980 study in which humans sitting under artificial, non-full spectrum light experienced a drain of energy and produced human stress hormones called ACTH (a hormone that stimulates steroid production in the adrenal gland cortex, also known as *adrenocorticotropin,* adversely affecting the liver and kidneys) and cortisol (an adrenal steroid too much of which can cause inflammation and autoimmune disease). These hormones also act as growth inhibitors and weaken immune system function.

Photobiolgist Dr. John N. Ott discovered through the time-lapse photographs he took for Walt Disney that distorted light and the harmful radiation it emits has an adverse and negative effect on plants, animals, and humans. "There is no question," he stated "that UV light in trace amounts, as in natural sunlight, acts as a life-supporting nutrient that is highly beneficial." UV light is what the skin, using cholesterols, converts into vitamin D, the immune vitamin, which reduces skin aging, and is imperative for immune system function. Dr. Ott, a pioneer in his field, believed light to be the missing link in curing cancer research. He wrote several excellent books on the subject and founded the Environmental Health and Light Research Institute in Tampa, Florida.

The pineal gland, regulated by sunlight signals sent through the retina of the eye, converts light signals into hormones, one of which is called melatonin, playing a large part in the function of sleep. Part of the recently uncovered role science has found in pineal/pituitary function is the production of more than thirty-six different hormones that account for brain and mental health, and overall hormone balance.

Pineal activity is also regulated by the earth's electromagnetic field, an important but poorly understood phenomenon. Distortion of atmospheric and electromagnetic energy (i.e. radiation through high voltage power lines, cell phones, micro waves, television/radio waves, etc.) causes distortion of the pineal's function, which therefore distorts the way perception, interpretation, and understanding of what is "seen" are experienced. Distorted perceptions trickle down into distorted digestion, immunity, circulation, respiration, elimination, reproductive function, body temperature, blood pressure, growth, motor function and all other human function cycles.

Our physics friend began to get the vision that in the same way raindrops separate out the individual colors visible from the white light of the sun, our human bodies, also prismatic conductors, separate white light into frequency spectrums and use those various colors to produce organic hormones. Since each color vibrates at a different frequency, not only are those frequencies interpreted by the pineal gland, but also by each of the 77 trillion cells of our bodies. Each frequency causes each aspect of the entire body to vibrate according to those frequencies. He already knew this, but then came the part that he hadn't studied. Some of these vibrations balance us and some of them take us out of balance; hormonally, emotionally, physically, mentally, digestively, and so forth. The proverbial light bulb went on in his head and he got it. He immediately understood that light could heal. He became an instantaneous supporter.

All this information can be charted as light spectrum energies that affect our emotions. When we have sufficient amounts of light and therefore balanced hormones, we are positively affected with mental, physical, spiritual, emotional, and sexual health. When we have insufficient amounts of light and there-

DOES THIS RELATE?

fore imbalanced hormones, we are negatively affected.

By way of introduction to the following chart it needs to be clear that light is transformed into hormones. Hormones serve both as fuel for organ function and as an e-motional (energy-motional) connector for the various "feeling" factors that cause us to think, understand, identify, choose, inspire, relate, balance, and create. When all light and hormone factors are optimal, the light centers of the body all connect, all systems fire, and health is achieved. The opposite takes place when they don't. See color insert, illustration 7.1.

> When all light and hormone **factors** are optimal, the light centers connect and health is **achieved**. The opposite takes place when they don't.

Raphaology:
the Revitalized Art
of Light Healing

"The great goal of life is living in agreement with nature."
ZENO 305 B.C.

WHEN WE THINK of light we think of sunlight, but we also think of artificial light — the light we get from lamps, flashlights, and other devices. We think of light for our convenience and tend to take sunlight for granted or, if we are influenced by marketing, we fear it. For purposes of clarity we will define light as pure waves of energy, without distortion, delivered in rays from the sun, carrying all the nutrients and minerals that make us feel whole. We will think of light as the ultimate healer.

> We will define **light** as pure waves of energy delivered in **rays** from the sun, carrying all the nutrients that make us whole. Think of light as the ultimate **healer**.

Each individual cell in our body is affected by light. Our eyes see by it, our hormones are made from it, our organs are fueled by it, our thoughts are motivated by it, and our emotions are impacted by it. Light and our relationship to it are among the most organic, sophisticated processes that exist. Our inter-relationship with light gives us the ability to heal and have permanent immunity to dis-ease. Through light we can allow our emotions to move through us, unblocking stagnancies as it goes and connecting us to every other living being. With light fully penetrated into us we feel the potential of universal information flowing through us. By utilizing this relationship with light in our daily lives, we no longer live in separation and lack and instead live in oneness and with the abundance of all there is, living to our full potential. Beyond the potential life force energy moving through you, you realize that potential force *is* you!

> Our inter-relationship with **light** gives us the ability to heal and have permanent **immunity** to dis-ease.

With awareness and respect, what you may have been taught about the order and colors of the human auric spectrum may vastly differ from what is used with Raphaology. Our practice of light spectrum does not fully agree with many of the traditional teachings about auras, chakras, rainbow spectrums, and the like. With that in mind, please take the following into consideration.

> New light relationships allow pure **crystallized** mineral energy to combine with physical matter producing the most pure **healing** available.

Due to the electromagnetic changes of the earth, gravitational resistance between energetic interactions, added to the collective awakening of consciousness on this planet, there are now new and different frequencies being absorbed and emitted by the whole universe—frequencies that end all traditions. We have entered the golden age. See color insert, illustration 8.1.

What may cause you to visually perceive the old colors of light, such as the rainbow, may be the distortion of light that occurs when light is actually bent or altered as it enters the altered electromagnetic field of the earth. The waves of light that move through the electro-magnetic field of earth's atmosphere are received by the eye's iris and retina and go directly to the pineal gland, which interpret these energy waves as colored light. When "seen" through one vibration, or frequency, they appear as one set of colors or light, and when viewed through another vibration or frequency of electromagnetism they are interpreted as another set of colors. The pattern of vibrations through which you are conditioned to interpret information will determine the colors that you "see" or perceive and interpret.

The light spectrum of colors we use in Raphaology is one that holds the frequencies that were not available many years ago. This new frequency pattern holds the least amount of distortion for today's world and can be used with more accuracy and efficacy. This peak frequency light holds the keys to restoring physical, mental, emotional, and light body health.

Light rays from the sun pour upon earth and all her inhabitants. We need them in their purest, most pristine form. Sunlight rays become distorted with the use of sunscreens on the skin, environmental pollution, modified foods, and technological interference. Any distortion in absorbed light alters its disbursement, absorption, utilization, and healing effects. The difference between adulterated and pure light is the difference between dis-ease and health. The crystallized minerals of the body are left lacking with distortion, but when charged with pure sun energy they positively affect our intelligence, our emotions, and our aging, vitality, and immunity.

ENZYMES

Light, energy, information, electricity, power, and color are all interchangeable terms because they are all differing aspects of the same thing. Another interchange can be added to those words: enzymes. The higher a food is in enzymes the higher levels of sunlight, energy, information, and power it contains. A medicinal plant that contains higher amounts of enzymes also contains higher amounts of energy and information to teach, train, remember, and guide your body to repairing and restoring itself.

> A **medicinal** plant that contains higher amounts of enzymes also contains higher amounts of energy and information to teach, train, remember, and guide your body to **repairing** and restoring itself.

Indigenous teachers and practitioners of ancient herbal traditions have held sacred the knowledge of the repairing aspects of herbal properties for complete healing by repairing, restoring, and maintaining every body function. In Raphaology, Jonathan's early findings, methodologies, and mastery were pooled with information gathered from tribes, nations and peoples that kept the ancient practices of true healing alive. By combining the best of the best and re-presenting ancient information and modern knowledge, Raphaology has formed a practical lifestyle of health wherein daily habits promote: repair of damage to the cellular body; balancing of hormones; restoration of all body functions; clearing of thoughts; and even regeneration of degenerated DNA, all for the purpose of unifying body, mind, emotions, and spirit.

> As a result of living with GMO foods, vaccines, chemically treated water, pharmaceutical toxins, and soil mineral **depletion,** we have become a world of people with extreme malnutrition.

While modern medicine may make it seem we are healthier than our ancestors, as a result of living with genetically modified organism (GMO) foods, vaccines, chemically treated water, pharmaceutical toxins, industrial waste, and soil mineral depletion we have actually become a world of people suffering from extreme malnutrition and weakened immune systems that make us susceptible to damaging pathogen invasion and host to their continued presence. Damage to our cells and chromosomes has occurred with each generation's consumption of contaminated food, drug, alcohol, air, water, and lifestyle pollutants leading us to what were once diseases of old age now being inflicted on the very young. But, there are ways for the earth, and us, to heal and return to peak health.

Raphaology combines the use of medicinal herbs with foods loaded with nutriceuticals for a **healing** combination unsurpassed by any other modality.

Peak Frequency Plant Therapy is the aspect of Raphaology that uses medicinal plants as herbs to repair damage in every aspect of the human body. We combine the use of medicinal herbs with foods loaded with nutriceuticals for a healing combination unsurpassed by any other modality.

<u>Herbs</u> **are plants that repair damage = phytoceuticals**
and
<u>Foods</u> **are plants that boost function = nutriceuticals**

HERBS

Herbs are two-fold: 1) concentrated taste sensations, spices, and variety for joyful living, and 2) nature's medicine. When used properly, medicinal herbs hold secrets, keys, and energetic information that can change your life for the better. Leaves and stems contain vital nutrients for the fueling of our organs and extremities. Berries, grains, and beans posses minerals that sustain and maintain quality of life. Roots and barks hold crucial elements for structure and strength. Flowers are acclimated toward the stars and planets of our universe and contain information about celestial organization and movement. Overall, specialized herbs provide the tools for maximum human healing.

When used properly medicinal **herbs** hold secrets, keys, and energetic information that can **change** your life for the better.

Specific herbs repair damage caused by bacteria, virus, parasites, acidity, malnourishment, and any other kind of degeneration. Medicinal herbs are the true healers of the plant world. As real medicine they receive and store vast amounts of particular kinds of sunlight that bring restoration of function to each organ. But organs do so much more than just perform physical body function. For instance, your brain is an organ that not only receives intelligence from the five senses but is also capable of forming thoughts from this intelligence, based on our will and intent. When we create our thoughts, instead of our thoughts creating us, we increase our consciousness, awareness, and are able to visualize our future. As the brain is exposed to more and more pure intelligence the thought/mind field increases, awareness grows, as do thoughts of our own creation, and experiential senses can become extrasensory and extraordinary.

As real medicine, herbs receive and store vast amounts of sunlight that bring **restoration** of function to each organ.

Herbs are what change the awareness of each specific organ. Yes, organs other than your brain have the ability to be aware, especially your heart. With growing awareness comes a growing capacity for each organ to improve its function. As each organ raises its capacity to receive and then give off greater amounts of light and information, each organ raises its frequency to perform at higher levels and your overall awareness, consciousness, and wellness increases. Each time the organ changes its capacity to raise its frequency, the function of that organ changes and allows more and more of you to express

> With growing **awareness** comes a growing capacity for each organ to improve its function.

yourself as your true self, your higher frequency self. If your frequency is growing constantly, your organ function will also change constantly, coming closer and closer to your capacity to be in consistent communication with your own experiential truth and with each other universal being. That's real health.

FOODS

Foods are the daily fruits of nature. Specific foods absorb specific colors of light from the sun, and like our bodies that transmute light into hormones, foods produce what are called enzymes, which are substances that boost and speed up the capacity and intensity for the body to function at its highest level. All natural foods contain some enzymes, but not all foods contain high enough enzymes to sustain your life force. *Peak Frequency Foods* contain surplus amounts of enzymes and nutrients that wake up and retrain the body and support our ability to truly live. As our bodies attain more true health they move closer to their true function and we move closer to our purpose of life, and become aware of reality through feeling memories of

> Enzymes are substances that **boost** and speed up the capacity and intensity for the body to **function** at its highest level.

how we are connected to all that is. *Peak Frequency Foods* boost this process and help us access our innate abilities and remember all our experiences.

To be more sensitive to your true self, and be able to recognize deceit more easily, eat foods of greater light, elevated enzymes, and higher frequency. Eating these foods gives the body the endurance to do what you have decided to do, the creativity to "see" how to do it, and the ability to achieve that high degree of super intelligence that you really need to be alive today.

Peak Frequency Foods contain surplus amounts of **enzymes** and **nutrients** that wake up and retrain the body and support our ability to truly live.

Most foods that have been presented to you as "healthy" have been marketed by a media that has something to sell you: their aim is to keep you in a state of half awareness so that you will continue buying and consuming what they have to sell. Take, for instance, the apple; "An apple a day keeps the doctor away" is a catchphrase that persuades you to eat apples. It has nothing to do with your health or keeping you from the doctor's office. In fact, it does the opposite. The apple overloads the gall bladder and liver functions, accelerates all pain processes, makes your body overly acidic, and in so doing, stimulates all inflammation and infection processes. In other words, an apple is far from an optimal food as are so many others you may have been led to believe are "healthy." A few of these other marketed foods are; oranges, carrots, celery, watermelon, iceberg lettuce, red and green peppers, green tea, grapefruit, chicken and eggs, cow's milk and cheese and ice cream products, pork (ham and bacon), shark, oats, rye, peanuts, walnuts, most squashes, processed sugars, white rice, yellow onions, parsley, black and white pepper, iodized table salt (including most sea salts), and peanut and canola oils.

Those foods do nothing to enhance your health. They have been genetically engineered and altered, keeping your body from operating efficiently. They will slow down your digestive process, in turn keeping you from gaining incoming information or finding self-knowledge. By eating these kinds of genetically modified and hybridized foods, you not only court disease, but you will stay stuck in the maze of your head that is recycled thoughts and media programming, all convincing you that you are what you have been programmed to be.

For the person who has been schooled on the evolving food pyramid and truly believes that in avoiding red meat, refined carbs, and fat they are eating healthfully, this can be difficult to absorb. So let's go further.

Most commercial foods have very little or no enzymes, rendering the food a "dead" food. These dead foods are highly marketed because there is more profit for manufacturers and grocers alike; their lifeless corpses last longer on the grocers shelves — representing less spoilage, less labor, and less turnover. Living foods support life; dead foods carry the power of death.

In short, you can eat foods that, at best, cause stagnation and at worst, dis-ease; or you can eat in ways that optimize your immunity, receptivity, clarity, and health.

INTERACTIVE DETERMINATION THERAPY

In Raphaology, the two dynamic natural healing components of herbs and foods are combined with a third component we call I.D. Therapy. Interactive Determination (ID) Therapy is a system of foot mapping that accesses the many nerve endings that form a path from the brain, continue the length of the body, and are attached to every single gland, organ, and system function along the way, ending on the feet. You may have heard of Reflexology, which is derived from ancient methods of connecting nerve meridians with its corresponding body part and stimulating the nerve

> ID Therapy is a **system** that accesses the many **nerve** endings from the brain, continue the length of the body, are attached to every gland, and organ **function** along the way, and ending on the feet.

ending to invoke healing. In a similar way, ID Therapy can detect light deficiencies, and their related imbalance and dysfunction, as well as determine what is needed to replace losses, repair damage, and restore and boost function. Jonathan, having lectured and taught in many mediums is best quoted with, "After many years of research and practice in the area of ID Therapy and working with the reflexive zones of the body, especially the feet, there is no doubt that this form of determining the cause of dysfunction and what is needed to repair or restore is one of the absolute most advanced medical diagnostic tools and healing methods there is, in many cases much more accurate than X-rays, laboratory tests, and modern medical technology."

Conjoining direct communication of the body's needs with the healing abilities of plants forms nature's true healing path: true medicine. Adding this together with the body's innate intelligence and ability to repair damage allows us our Creator-given ability to use every physical and energetic element for our health and well-being. Through receiving the gifts of our earth mother we obtain true health, and once we have attained our radiant health, we can help her achieve her peak frequency as a sun. But where is the science in that?

Science versus Art

"Science is built up of facts, as a house is built up of stones; but an accumulation of facts is no more science than a heap of stones is a house."
POINCARE IN SCIENCE AND HYPOTHESIS

WHERE DID SCIENCE COME FROM and why do we seem to place more importance on science than art? Perhaps we can agree that art is the imitation of nature by the use of man's various means of expression and adaptation, and science is the interpretation of nature using man's perceptions, theories, measurements, tests, and synthetic elements. In ancient days societies lauded, provided for and protected its artists, while current trends acclaim, fund and protect its sciences. Is science the new art?

Science began as postulations, theories, and con-

> Art is the imitation of nature by the use of man's **expression** and adaptation, and science is the interpretation of nature using man's **perceptions**, measurements, and synthetic elements.
> Is science the new **art**?

jectures of how nature works by observing and forming conceptual theories on those observations using common sense and linear logic, and then forming repeatable tests that would produce a consistent result as proof that the theory is correct, no matter how the test and its elements were skewed to obtain the repeatable result. Science may or may not be an accurate account of the true formation or function of natural elements because it seeks to use unnatural means to prove its theoretic observations of nature.

Art began as the imitation of nature without theory or postulation, simply reproduction for the pure intent and enjoyment of imitating what nature does, adapted to the genre whether drawn, painted, written, danced, sung, textiled, or articulated. Art often uses natural components to imitate certain aspects of the whole of nature, while science seeks to separate each component of nature and uses the individual component to explain the whole. If each part of the whole were the same as the whole it could not be broken down into differing parts, therefore any one part cannot explain the whole. Science looks at anything that it has not taken the time to observe and classify as anecdotal and therefore unscientific. Nature is definitely unscientific.

> **Science** looks at anything that it has not taken the time to observe and classify as anecdotal and therefore unscientific. **Nature** is definitely unscientific.

Science has led man to believe that he can quantify, reproduce, and refine nature with better results. Since science uses man-made mediums, capable of measuring only what it can observe, science is limited to man's perceptive abilities. By believing what is scientific we are limited by the scope of scientific explanation. Take for instance the Middle Ages, during which science told man that the world was flat—and it was believed there was an edge from which to fall into oblivion. People tend not to venture into what they believe to be impossible. And this mindset negates exploration. In the past, science has served to separate humanity from humanity by virtue of its limited ability to observe the whole picture. So, where would we be if someone had not exclaimed for all to hear that the world was round? And if someone had not believed this and ventured forth?

There currently exists two basic schools of thought, or two models of perceiving nature. One is associated with Western scholarship — i.e. knowledge acquired using methods based in physical evidence, experimentation, and measurement. The other model is associated with the Eastern approach — i.e. knowledge received from an external source through esoteric means in a state of meditation. Esoteric knowledge is not something acquired. It is considered a sharing of universal experience.

The Western approach, based in material components, is slow, complicated, and linear, while the Eastern approach is rapid; almost immediate, simple, and multi-dimensional. Following the Western route, it has taken over a thousand years to arrive at a level of knowledge that was common in the East over three millennia ago. Modern medicine would be considered a Western concept, while Raphaology would be included as an Eastern approach.

Raphaology is a healing art. Modern medicine is a marketed science. Commercial medicine deals in the science of invasive tests, harsh procedures, and often brutal measures to separate out one or more components for the purpose of diagnosing and treating symptoms, which are then often treated with synthetic medications. The treatment of symptoms alone disassociates the symptom within

> Raphaology is a **healing** art. Modern **medicine** is a marketed science.

you from you as a whole. Symptoms are the body's reaction to the presence of malnutrition, acidity, toxicity, pathogens, deficiency, dysfunction or damage. Separating the symptoms and viewing them as disconnected entities justifies the use of harsh chemicals and invasiveness against the symptom, leaving you as a whole more injured and still dis-eased. This method of treatment has little to do with healing. Healing through the ages has always been considered an art form, and science is modern man's way of defining it. Since man has not been able to best nature in healing, man's science has served to diagnose, control, and treat symptoms of disease with synthesized forms of the natural medicines that truly cure, convincing you that because science doesn't deal in cures, no cure exists.

> The treatment of symptoms alone disassociates the **symptom** within you from you as a whole.

Many have asked over the years "Where is the science that proves Raphaology works?" While science can be used to explain how Raphaology Medicine works, science cannot replicate what Raphaology does. Science also cannot explain how or why the human body works, merely some aspects of what it does.

> While science can be used to explain how **Raphaology** medicine works, science cannot replicate what Raphaology does.

Modern medicine as it exists today began only a few hundred years ago. *It* is really the "alternative" to the medicine that has been practiced for thousands of years by our ancestors. Indigenous people with the knowledge of healing arts are respected and honored as healers, given the titles of shamans, sages, etc., in the same way that modern medical science titles its authorities as doctors.

The body *always* wants to heal itself. There is a database of spontaneous remissions and spontaneous recoveries, particularly from critical conditions such as cancer, but if science

hasn't discovered this aspect of us yet, are you going to remain in the Dark Ages and limit your spontaneous healing
abilities to science's limited view?

Medicine's Modern Origins

"Medicine is a collection of uncertain prescriptions
the result of which, taken collectively,
are more fatal than useful to mankind."

NAPOLÉON BONAPARTE 1798

MODERN MEDICAL DOCTORS have their roots in grave digging. Less than a few hundred years ago there was very little "scientific" knowledge about the human body and it was thought that if bodies and their various parts could be studied up close and personal more advancement could be made in medicine. Since science and chemistry had not advanced enough to cut up, experiment on, and examine living humans, the recently departed were often secretly exhumed, their organs and various parts removed for study, and the remains were returned to their graves. While it is true that this process enabled the grave poaching scientists to explore and learn more about the human body, it was still the study of dead body parts, with unknown dis-easement, leaving science with only theory as to how those parts might work under healthy living conditions.

Modern medical science as a whole still bases its diagnosis, treatment, drugs, and protocols on the information collected from dis-eased and dead bodies. The findings—from non-living, unhealthy, separated samples under clinical conditions with controlled environments, using synthetic chemicals to produce specific results—do not provide the living human body with what it needs for health or can safely use. The use of modern medicine's drugs, surgeries, radiations, and cytotoxins (cell poisons) to treat symptoms do more to harm, violate, damage, degenerate, and traumatize the whole body while ignoring its innate healing process. It remains more barbaric and invasive than anything it accuses indigenous healers of practicing. Natural healing arts can intervene in critical situations with the use of gentle, but highly effective life-supporting herbs and energies, and hands-on comforting that infuse life without trauma.

Modern medicine does have a place. Surgery, drugs, and invasive **treatments** can save one's life in an emergency.

This is not to suggest that modern medicine does not have its place. There are many instances where surgical procedures, drugs, and invasive treatments can save one's life in an emergency. But these critical situations are too often looked upon as a permanent condition that remains for the rest of the individual's life, driving the doctors to tell a patient that he or she must evermore take the same prescription that was required during crisis measures. Once crisis is over, let that harrowing experience inspire the individual to make changes in his or her lifestyle that will promote healing

Once crisis is over, let that **experience** inspire the individual to make changes that will promote **healing** and prevent the body from developing conditions that lead to crisis.

and prevent the body from developing conditions that will ever lead to crisis again.

Modern science and the commercialized medicine that emanates from it do NOT study healing or prevention of dis-ease. Most medical professionals do not study nutritional elements and are instead taught that while some food, taken in excess, can be at the root of some disorders, overall it is irrelevant to healing. They are taught how to diagnose symptoms and treat the symptoms of dis-ease with pharmaceuticals until a surgery is required to remove or replace the damaged or debilitated part. They do know that nutritional elements can actually prevent dis-ease from forming, but they are not schooled in any particulars.

There are men and women of knowledge and integrity who have made and continue to make vast strides in learning the living body, how it works, what it needs to heal, and what natural elements safely assist the process. Beside, Jonathan, there are two other men in recent times that stand out as greats who have contributed more substantially to the true understanding and healing of the human body than all the men of commercial medicine put together. But you will probably never hear about them on the 6:00 news or read about them in newspapers or history books.

ROYAL RAYMOND RIFE

Dr. Royal Raymond Rife, a pleomorphic cellular biochemist, discovered that specific frequencies of light can heal every life-threatening condition in the human body. Dr. Rife was able to observe spectrum frequencies destroying harmful antibodies with the use of the world's most powerful microscope that he built back in the early 1930s. He studied Zeis optics in Germany and developed his powerful magnification microscope using natural quartz crystal optics, dark fields, and cold light with the ability to study *living* cycles of microbial cells, bacteria, virus and fungus. His sophisticated technology remains more advanced than any modern scientific equipment used today.

Dr. Rife's passionate interest in microbes led him to study and then classify each microbial antibody with a "Mortal Oscillatory Rate" (MOR), cataloging each one with a frequency, light spectrum vibration, and the low auditory frequency that would literally kill and disintegrate the antibody within the body of its human host, thereby killing cancer, tuberculosis, typhus, and many other life-threatening microbes without harsh chemicals, surgery, or any discomfort whatsoever.

Dr. Rife also developed and manufactured frequency equipment called the "Rife Ray Machine" that was used with 100 percent efficacy in many terminal cancer treatment hospitals and clinics, including the University of Southern California (USC), in the 1930s, literally putting an end to cancer. Making the national headlines of almost every major newspaper across the country, Dr. Rife was celebrated and lauded as a national hero, liberating the world of cancer. Due to greed, lawsuits, the death of Dr. Milbank Johnson, its largest mainstream supporter, and the ensuing lack of funds, Dr. Rife's technology was obscured and the newly developed penicillin took its place in the media. Penicillin claimed to wipe out bacteria, but it eventually created new super resistant bacteria, while becoming the excuse for pharmaceutical companies to claim their victory over bacterial infection. This left cancer and other viruses at the mercy of laboratories funded by chemical companies, medical associations, and agencies whose job it is to ensure profit for their stockholders, chairmen, presidents, and investors. And there is limited profit in curing dis-ease.

HANS JENNY

A Swiss by the name of Hans Jenny, a forerunner in the field of vibrational research, discovered that sound frequencies produce a restoration of proper form, thereby eliminating disease. His unique observational approach to monitoring and categorizing the effects that vibrations in their different frequencies produce is remarkable. Physicality is unarguably made up of matter and vibration. It is virtually the living vibratory pulsations of our light/energy body that provides the dynamic for the material that we call our physical bodies to come to life, grow, and heal.

The basics of new vibrational observations, which he coined "Cymatics," had Hans Jenny studying wave phenomenon, vibrational effects, harmonic oscillations and their structures, kinetics, and dynamics, all performed with repeatable success to demonstrate that vibration is the unified force of Creation. Using various mediums he broadcast and penetrated these mediums with sound vibrations and was able to literally recreate every single form in nature, including plant life and the organs, cells, and bones of the human body. When he applied these same corresponding tonal frequencies to the various parts of the body, each body part that had sustained any damage began to repair itself when its original frequency was run through its structural field.

Mr. Jenny knew that logical science had long been of the estimation that the whole consists of the component parts, and that observing the individual parts gives the whole picture, therefore rendering it unnecessary to be concerned with the whole. He knew this would be true *if* we had the power of truly comprehensive observation, and this is exactly what he sought to acquire. His vibrational healing methods cured the "scientifically incurable" dis-eases with little more than a few vibrations.

Rife was able to see with his powerful microscope the vibratory rates of harmful antibodies and discern the frequencies that would kill them while not harming any living human cells. Jenny was able to recreate the cellular structure of living human tissue, as well as the harmful pathogens with the use of frequency tones, eliminating pathogens safely and painlessly.

JONATHAN: THUNDER: WOLF

A pure-blooded Scandinavian Viking Jonathan: Thunder: Wolf, founder, professor, and doctor of Raphaology medicine, self-healing master and professor of cellular light dynamics, was able to discern the frequencies of plants and to relate their complementary healing frequency to the exact rate of recurrence of each human organ and tissue for their application in restoring vibrational health. He has dedicated his life to the study and practice of light medicine with the discerning capability of applying specific plants that can both restore vibrational balance and neutralize, annihilate, and remove the source of damage without harm, trauma, or violation to its human host.

LIVING MATTER AS VIBRATING FORM

As living matter, defined by the materials and vibrational patterns that govern our human form, our bodies are more profound, more intangible, more dynamic than any science can ever come close to copying or defining. Even if science cannot agree, we are literally formed by combinations of vibrations, differing frequency rates, that cause us to vary one from another, resulting in how we look, sound, feel, and heal. We function wholly within the dynamics that govern our vibratory end limits. If science ever accepts this, I hope it is something it never seeks to control.

We can control our form, and thus our deformities, by changing our thinking processes to more positive and creative ones, by changing our words to higher frequencies that promote happier, more pleasurable expressions that will help change the very vibration that determines our state of mental, emotional, physical, and spiritual well being. Our words are the vibrational expression of who we are, what we are, how we are, and why we are.

> When we understand and work with the **biorhythms** of our own bodies we become the masters of self-manifestation, and are immune to every invading **vibration** that is not in harmony with us..

Modern science teaches us to believe only what we can see and to fear what is unseen or can't be seen, yet it uses technology that purposefully does not "see" living matter. Because of this fear of the unknown and the unexplainable, science gives us cause to exist in fear and to have no trust in our innate abilities, acting on the "what if" principle. "What if" is the theory that guides the scientific view of dis-ease because if one does not "see" what is causing it one cannot "see" how to cure it or to repair it without invasion. So "what if" science cannot cure? Then it favors controlling the disease symptoms with drugs, with you as its dependant customer, creating a seemingly slower progression of degeneration until it's time to remove or replace the problematic source in a surgical procedure. Scientific medicine would have us rely on academic professionals to control our symptoms, with the belief that we are incapable of healing ourselves. And with the debilitating fear of "what if" we are unable to heal ourselves, then science offer us its only option: use cumulatively harmful drugs to control the symptoms.

Since science has been unable to pinpoint the components required for health or for a disease-free body, it adds incomplete, synthetic vitamins to the diet and hopes some of your body's needs are being met. This is not the healing answer. The Food and Drug Administration (FDA) would have us believe that the Recommended Daily Value (RDV) of vitamins and minerals is the same for every individual. They suggest a pitifully low dosage is enough to sustain good health for each and every person, along with the representation that synthetic nutrients can be substituted for organic, while ignoring the destructive side effects caused by their use. Please note that in the 1990s, the director of the FDA died around the age of forty from a common malnutrition problem.

Modern science would have us be afraid of herbs due to their possible toxicity, while they continue to administer potential-

> Modern science would have us be afraid of herbs due to their possible **toxicity**, while they continue to administer potentially deadly **toxins** in controlled amounts.

ly deadly toxins in controlled amounts. There are some toxic herbs, which are not used in healing, yet all pharmaceuticals are potentially toxic. The FDA, medical doctors, and scientists know this and rush to inform you of the side effects of each drug, but offer you the security that they will test for and monitor the damage that will expectedly occur to liver, kidneys, or heart so that when critical levels accumulate they will be happy to rush you into surgery to remove, replace, or invasively repair the damage.

Abandoning our health to "professional" medical treatment has proven that despite the sixty-year "war on cancer," the billions of dollars and man hours expended, and the success of alternative therapies, modern medicine has yet to develop a way to cure this disease. Matthias Rath M.D., having achieved success in natural biomedical cancer elimination, says "A consequence of the war against cancer has been the military-like approach to treating those who have been stricken. Conventional cancer treatments involve attacking cancer cells with lethal chemicals, devastating radiation, and dangerous surgery. These methods indiscriminately destroy both diseased and healthy cells. Even when patients are able to survive such harsh therapies, the struggle for health often becomes continuous as their weakened bodies develop new diseases or tumors." Add to this the fact that once metastasis (the spread of cancer) occurs, modern medicine is helpless to stop it and therefore the high rate of death keeps climbing for patients who pursue commercial treatment.

Borrowing some words from Jethro Kloss' 1939 work, *Back to Eden*, "Nature has provided a remedy for every disease that might afflict us, there is no disease for which nature has not provided a remedy. Our scientists and medical colleges have failed to find the 'true remedies' found in nature, for if they did, then poisonous drugs and chemicals would be eliminated and sickness would be rare indeed." He further states, "Men who violate the natural laws of health are ignorant of the relation of the laws of living (eating, drinking, resting, working, pure water, air, sunshine, and nature's herbs and foods), until they have some kind of sickness or illness, they do not realize their own condition is caused by violating these laws. If they realized their unnatural conditions as the cause of their illness, then they would know that returning to nature would restore the body to its original health."

Even though we may know better, the way most of us exercise our common sense about health is to rush to the drugstore or our M.D. when we have an allergy attack, headache, constipation, infection, pain, or upset stomach. We have been conditioned that we shouldn't have to suffer any pain, and we can easily stop pain by taking a pill that will take care of the problem; a pill for every ill. We have begun to think that our problem is cured just because we don't feel the symptom anymore. Common sense ought to tell us that if we have pain there is a problem. It's telling us to fix the problem so the pain can naturally go away as a result of the problem being resolved. Should you cut yourself and let that cut stay dirty, infection would set in. Swelling and bacterial damage occurs, and pain would worsen, leading to worse conditions, and you would not expect that wound to heal. You would never leave a visible gash full of dirt and bacteria, take a pain pill, and hope for the best. But because our internal dirt and infection are not visible, we think we can just mask the pain and the problem is taken care of. Nothing could be further from the truth.

Medical doctors, those who are brilliant diagnosticians with the ability to intuitively interpret information that results

> We have been **conditioned** that we shouldn't have to suffer any pain, and can stop pain by taking a pill that takes care of the **problem**; a pill for every ill.

> **Common** sense ought to tell us that if we have pain there is a **problem**.

from the various tests and technologies that it has contrived to "see" inside the body, are exercising their artistic aspect, and when pressed with an answer that science and medicine cannot provide, will admittedly say "when it comes down to answers, medicine is really an art."

Jonathan's and my mission is to inform and assist everyone who is so inclined to take full accountability for their individual health and get to know their bodies; what they put in it; how to repair and heal it; and how to stay immune to the perpetual onslaught of invaders that we all live with. Nature is still the best medicine, and its healing practices are the art that keeps us free of dis-ease.

> **Nature** is still the best medicine, and its healing **practices** are the art that keeps us free of dis-ease.

We Are Not Victims of Disease

"There is no medicine like hope, no incentive so great, and no tonic so powerful as expectation of something tomorrow."

ORLSON SWETT MARDEN 1910

EVERY SINGLE ILLNESS, including cancer, is not just something that happens to us, something that is beyond our control. Even though we may hate to admit it, we are completely accountable for every disease that occurs inside our bodies. We create it, we control it, and we can get rid of it. We are in charge of our bodies: what we put into them, the thoughts they think, the feelings they feel, the decisions they make, their responses or reactions, the relationships they choose, and what they produce. We are only victims if we think, react, feel, and decide that we are. When we are not victims all our thoughts, intentions, responses, feelings, actions, relationships, and creations are powerful, truthful, full of integrity, and, most of all, free of the blaming and victim mentality.

> We are only **victims** if we think, react, feel, and decide that we are.

The current way of thinking about germs, which has people believing we are victims of nasty germs and are helpless against them, is convenient for the medical business. This belief prompts us to seek out professional medical help to rid ourselves of destroying buggers, medical assistance which yet creates further environs in which more buggers can live. WE are *not* helpless bystanders when it comes to germs. We live with germs on a daily basis. As a matter of fact, almost 80 percent of our systems depend on germs of one form or another to help us digest, transport fluids and waste, and have immunity to other germs. It is when the organic balance inside us gets out of balance, or we host invasions of external antibody pathogens, that germs become hazardous. We are ultimately responsible for the internal environment of our bodies that cause the imbalances that create dis-ease and form life threatening conditions.

> We can **prevent** over 90 percent of all dis-ease by recognizing conditions that are causing **toxicity** to build up and get rid of them.

We can prevent over 90 percent of all dis-ease by recognizing what conditions are present in the digestive system that are causing toxicity to build up and getting rid of them. Internal acids, toxins, dehydration, oxygen deprivation, vitamin and mineral deficiencies provide the host environment for bacterium and virus to live, grow, and proliferate. Their resulting symptoms have been named such things as high cholesterol, diabetes, heart disease, and cancer. Changing what we are putting in our bodies that cause these conditions is what prevents

> Changing what we put in our bodies to cause these **conditions** prevents dis-ease. Knowing the foods to change conditions that host **dangerous** antibodies and the herbs that destroy them is the cure.

dis-ease. Knowing the proper foods to change conditions that host dangerous antibody growth and the specific herbs that destroy them is how we practice the cure.

After experiencing first hand and witnessing countless people overcome dis-ease by changing foods, supplements, liquids, lifestyle, thinking, and feelings it has become readily apparent to me that cleaning out the internal toxicity eliminates the environment that harmful germs depend on for their existence and growth. The germ theory denies the power within, which ignores the ability to respond favorably to our lives and change the physiological and psychological responses or habits that are polluting our internal organs. Remember that every dis-ease starts in the digestive system and is caused primarily by toxic internal environments that

> Every dis-ease starts in the digestive system and is caused by toxic **internal** environments that produce malfunction and malnutrition, and we are responsible for those **conditions**.

produce congestion, acidity, damage, blockage, malfunction, malnutrition, and mutation, and we are responsible for those internal conditions by virtue of the quality of our foods, our stresses, our emotions, our attitude, and the like, which provide the host environment for excessive "germ" presence and proliferation.

GERM THEORY VERSUS TOXICITY THEORY

The germ theory goes like this: "germs make us sick." The germ theory was postulated to imply that we are not responsible for dis-ease; that dis-ease is imposed upon us from a germ source, and it is those germs that make us sick. This convenient theory implies that germs can be treated and controlled with pharmaceutical-grade antibiotics and inhibitors, and thus encourages the use of medicine for financial profit from controlling your illness through symptom management and treatment.

This germ theory implies that the internal conditions of the body have nothing to do with the hosting and proliferation of harmful germs.

Let's look at a simile of germs and toxins, comparing it to flies and garbage. Germs in our simile are like flies, and toxicity is like garbage. If you were to have a pile of ever-growing garbage in your yard, the pile of rotting and putrefying garbage would begin to draw flies and host their reproduction. The larger the pile of garbage the more flies it would support. When you remove the garbage a phenomenal thing happens: the flies go away to find another garbage pile they can live in. When you remove the toxins in your body, which is the real sickness, the germs have nowhere to live and they go away, too.

A healthy body and immune system consists of the ability to constantly recognize and remove these germs, no matter how many, or what kind they may be. While conversely, a toxic and dysfunctional body and immune system is dumbed down, slowed down, and has debilitated white blood cells that are powerless against the pathogenic germs and rendered incapable of removing the excess toxins in which they live.

Three reasons why the germ theory is devastating are:

1. It encourages harmful habits by suggesting that it doesn't matter what we eat, think, or do; we are all going to be attacked by germs or carcinogens and there is nothing we can do to stop it.

2. It encourages people to accept that doctors must use costly, harsh, damaging and sometimes deadly drugs and treatments to rid their body of these germs or their degenerative symptoms.

3. It encourages the denial that the human body has the intelligence or ability to repair and heal itself.

By accepting this germ theory we open our physical body to a virtual reality of antibody acceptance and a dis-empowering belief that we are intrinsically incapable of improving our conditions of health, lifestyle, or decisions.

It is by receiving new information, higher intelligence, and appropriate tools that we become capable of making new decisions and acting on them for phenomenal changes that better our lives and health. Knowing a new concept provides another choice and different actions that can be taken. Removing drugs, especially antibiotics and vaccines; eliminating chlorinated and fluorinated water; avoiding air pollution; abstaining from household cleaning and cosmetic toxins and pesticides; pushing away from processed, refined, microwaved, and mineral-deficient foods; staying away from unnatural chemicals, additives, and hormones in foods; and replacing harmful emotions with positive and courageous ones; along with new foods and herbal remedies, will begin to correct the damage that has already occurred.

Whether your goal is to be healthier, feel sexier, have more intelligence, lose weight, get stronger, feel more confident, communicate better, sleep deeper, deal with stress easier, or be happier, we all achieve these goals in the same manner: the proper care and feeding of our human bodies. Each of us has the same basic physiology to deal with, with a few differences, like DNA, metabolic cycles, and blood types. There are blood type diets, which hold some merit but include protein and fat factors that conform more to science than the body's natural organic tendencies. There are diets of many varieties, accessed in print, on television, in practical trials, and by word of mouth. But few are based on how our bodies actually use, digest, and metabolize nutrients. Most marketed diets conform to the intake of calories, proteins, fats, fibers, and carbohydrates based on the science of sterile and chemical laboratory findings and have little to do with actual health, relying more on immediate gratification with hidden ramifications.

Why Medical Doctors Don't Recommend Vitamin Therapy

"One of the first duties of the physician is to educate the masses not to take medicine. A good physician treats the disease: the great physician treats the patient who has the disease."

WILLIAM OSLER 1889

WHEN NUTRIENTS ARE TESTED by medical science as therapy they use very low and varied doses — so clinical reports show ambiguous results. Erratic and varied results are not proof of efficacy and are therefore disregarded. Without knowing exactly what nutrients the human body requires for individual function or overall health, medical science is baffled by correct amounts. What science can't explain, it prefers to ignore. Because uncertainty prevails, they opt to err on the side of caution, so recommended nutritional dosages fail to meet even minimal health standards. For this and other reasons most medical doctors don't study or concern themselves with nutrition as a form of treatment.

In the scientific and pharmaceutical world, the prevailing theory is "one drug for every one disease." While this theory may serve the drug world that strives to cite more symptoms for which to develop more drugs, it is definitely not true for the world of nutrients. There are only a few dozen nutrients, yet in the body those few nutrients sponsor countless organic chemical reactions. Anything that is vitamin- or mineral-based will produce multiple reactions, confounding the best of scientists. They refuse to accept that a single nutrient can produce such a vast array of beneficial results:

Vitamin A
Antioxidant
Anticarcinogen
Keeps eyes and mucous membranes moist
Supports and increases respiration
Repairs cells
Increases brain hormones
Supports sleep cycles
Converts proteins into tissue
Boosts T-cells in thymus gland
Promotes pineal function
Sight in light and dark
Healthy supplements range from 20,000 - 100,000 IU daily

B-Complex Vitamins
Anti-acid
Antibacterial
Anticarcinogen
Immune booster and regulator
Relieves back aches and headaches
Digestion enhancement
Decreases depression
Increases adrenal function
Improves insulin production
Balances metabolism
Reduces stress
Protects nerves

Produces red blood cells
Increases bone density
Creates hormones
Organically synthesizes RNA and DNA
Healthy supplements range from 2,000 - 40,000 mg daily

Vitamin C
Antitoxin
Antihistamine
Antiviral
Regulates blood sugar
Elevates mood and depression
Increases immunity
Repairs blood vessels and arteries
Breaks up cholesterol
Mobilizes iron in blood
Converts cholesterol into bile
Forms collagen
Metabolizes carbohydrates
Healthy supplements range from 2,000 - 20,000 mg daily

Vitamin D
Powers immune system
Metabolizes calcium
Deposits calcium into bones and teeth
Prevents osteoporosis and osteomalacia
Strengthens muscles
Prevents anemia
Prevents rickets
Healthy supplements range from 2,000 - 10,000 I.U. daily

Vitamin E
Antioxidant
Heart disease therapy
Heals burns
Reduces epilepsy and seizures

Prevents heart attack and stroke
Increases fertility and sexual potency
Heals nerves and their disorders
Reduces and breaks up blood clots
Tones muscles
Heals scars
Produces anti-bodies
Supports adrenals and pituitary glands
Reduces cataracts and arthritis
Healthy supplements range from 800 - 8,000 IU daily

By examining just a few of the above nutrients amidst the complete complement and their involvement in the formative and curative functions within the human body, it is easy to see the confusion. How can so few nutrients assist and perform so many processes in so many areas? It is because those nutrients combine with many other enzymes, oxygen, fluids, hormones, and microbial organisms to perform the countless mechanical, metabolic, and meteoric functions that sustain life. Because we are all uniquely different in our needs, deficiencies, stresses, healing factors, lifestyles, and habits we all require differing nutrients and amounts at various times under a variety of conditions. There is NO set amount for daily requirements that applies to everyone.

There is a great misnomer among medical scientists that if nutrients are therapeutic they must be dangerous because therapeutic drugs are dangerous. Nothing could be farther from the truth. Their theory is that organic elements are equal to inorganic elements, which has prompted agencies that now seek to control and police nutritional supplements. Please take a stand and consider opposing the regulation of nature's nutrients.

The recommended amount of vitamin C by the FDA is 200 mg, enough to prevent scurvy (blood vessel damage), yet we still see scurvy on a daily basis; they just changed the name. Now it's called atherosclerosis (hardening of the arteries). Stress alone depletes the water soluble C and the B-complex vitamins, rendering the daily *minimal* amount of vitamin C at 2,000 mg to keep scurvy from forming, and more to prevent atherosclerosis. Even more is needed if you live in the city, endure chronic stress, eat poor quality food, and are subjected to industrial or environmental pollutants or pesticides.

We cannot deprive our cells of nutrition for long without having to pay for it at some point. Specific malnutrition produces specific deficiency symptoms. Twenty-six percent of patients discharged from hospitals are more malnourished than when they went in; especially after eating white bread and Jello™ (common hospital fare). Isn't it interesting that 80-90 percent of the reason that caused them to get hospitalized was their poor state of nutrition. Eating the proper daily doses of nutrients will prevent dis-ease, and supplementation of large enough doses of nutrients will cure dis-ease. Commercial medicine has made us afraid of too high of doses of nutrients, therefore making us afraid of taking any at all. Ten people have died in the past five years of vitamin overdose. Some 106,000 died in the year 2009 from pharmaceutical overdose.

> Ten people have died in the past five years of **vitamin** overdose. Some 106,000 died in the year 2009 from **pharmaceutical** overdose.

Because the lack of one single nutrient can produce so many dis-eases, the supplementation of a single nutrient can cure so many dis-eases. Nutrition heals all dis-eases. If you have high blood pressure, high cholesterol, cancer, diabetes, and fibromyalgia simultaneously—all problems disappear by healing any one of them. In the organic body, you can't heal one dis-ease and keep the others. By nourish-

> Because the lack of one single **nutrient** can produce so many dis-eases, the **supplementation** of a single nutrient can cure so many dis-eases.

ing the body, you provide it with the tools to fix all the problems. Nutrients, not drugs, enable the body to heal itself. Not one cell in the human body is made of a drug, but every cell is made up of nutrients.

In the 1920s Max Gerson M.D. and nutritionist said, "It's the doctors duty to activate the body's own healing mechanism." At the time Dr. Gerson was having a better than 50 percent cure rate with terminally ill cancer patients, compared to the less than 30 percent cure rate that commercial medicine has today with non-terminal cancer patients. Since it is illegal today in the U.S. to treat or cure cancer with anything other than radiation, surgery, and chemotherapy, many people and some smart doctors use Dr. Gerson's, and other nutritional therapies to cure cancer in countries outside the U.S.

> Nutrients, not drugs, enable the **body** to heal itself. Not one cell in the human body is made of a drug, but every **cell** is made up of nutrients.

- Dr. Linus Pauling, winner of two Nobel Peace Prizes, was curing the common cold in the 1930s with high doses of vitamin C. He took 20,000 mg vitamin C daily and was out riding his horse on the range at over ninety years of age when the doctors that poo-pooed his principles were long dead.
- Dr. Fred R. Klenner in the 1940s was curing all viral diseases with high doses of vitamin C.
- Dr. Dean Ornish cures cardiovascular disease with nutrition, stress reduction and meditation, and without the use of drugs, surgery, or invasive measures.
- Dr. Matthias Rath cures cancers with nutrition, amino acids, anti-oxidants, immune stimulating vitamins and minerals, and oxygen.

Food supplements to reduce stress and cure dis-ease are safer, cheaper, and more effective in curing all dis-ease, yet commercial medicine continues to treat malnutrition symptoms with drugs.

Healing Symptoms

*"Those who think they have no time for healing
will sooner or later have to find the time for illness."*
EDWARD STANLEY 1893

THE SYMPTOMS OF HEALING occur when the instinctive powers of the body begin exchanging something of poor quality for something better. When superior quality goods replace inferior quality elements the body naturally expels the poor elements through its detoxification channels; lungs, colon, skin, and kidneys. This detoxification process may produce skin rashes, bad breath, diarrhea, body odor, headaches, itching, acne, and the like. Healing symptoms are telling you that your body is expelling the bad and replacing it with good. If your intent is for healing, do NOT stop this process. Consider that you are making an easy-payment plan now toward the purchase of health, instead

> The symptoms of **healing** occur when the instinctive powers of the body begin exchanging something of poor **quality** for something better.

of a giant balloon payment of critical disease or death at the end of forty to fifty years.

In some cases, colds or even fevers, which haven't appeared for a long time, may now appear. THIS IS NATURE'S WAY OF HOUSECLEANING! Understand these actions are constructive, even though uncomfortable. We need NEVER try to stop these symptoms with the use of drugs. Using over-the-counter drugs or going to a medical doctor at this point would result in a prescription that would inhibit healing, adding more inferior elements to further toxify the body as well as keeping the fleeing toxins trapped, causing further degeneration. These are neither deficiency conditions nor allergic manifestations. In actuality, any kind of illness is a result of toxins being thrown off by the body in its effort to heal itself and the symptoms of fever, diarrhea, vomiting, rashes, etc., should not be stopped (except in extreme or prolonged cases), but rather eased with herbal teas or extracts, or the toxins will remain in the body. You may certainly use herb medicine to assist detoxification and relieve symptoms such as thyme for fever; chamomile for rashes, cramps, and vomiting; sarsaparilla for diarrhea or food poisoning; and noni or American ginseng for energy.

> Any kind of **illness** is a result of toxins being thrown off by the body in its effort to **heal** itself.

We have been taught very little about the relationship between the quality of food we consume and recovery from illness. The higher the food enzyme content, the quicker we will recover from disease. When illness sets in use the fruits starting with the letter "P" from the *Peak Frequency Food* list (Appendix A) and watch remarkable things begin to happen to the body as well as the mind! The amazing intelligence present in every single cell of the body

> The higher the food **enzyme** content, the quicker we will **recover** from disease.

and its innate ability to function efficiently immediately becomes manifest. The rule may be stated as follows:

When the food coming into the body is of higher quality than the tissues of which the body is made, the body begins to discard the lower grade materials and tissues to make room for the superior materials — which is used to make new and healthier tissue.

The "P" fruits—papaya, pineapple, pear, plum, red potato, persimmon, passion fruit, and pomegranate provide the highest quality enzymes and nutrients with which to begin the healing process.

When we suddenly stop the use of toxic stimulants such as acidic coffee or soda (especially cola drinks), headaches are common and a letdown can occur. This is due to the discarding of toxins, which are removed from the tissue and transported through the blood stream during many bodily cycles. Before the noxious agents reach their final point of elimination, these irritants register as pain; in other words, a headache. When we feel lower energy, it is due to the slower action of the heart—the resting phase, which is different from the artificial stimulation of more rapid heart action forced upon the body by food poisons (stimulants such as refined sugar). The previous more rapid heart rate produced a feeling of exhilaration, and now the slower action produces a state of mind, which can easily be interpreted as depression. Within three days, however, the symptoms usually vanish and the recuperation, which follows will leave us feeling stronger.

Accepting accountability for the conditions in your current life situation, whether those conditions are creative or destruc-

> Accepting accountability for the conditions in your current life **situation**, whether those conditions are creative or destructive, is the first step to **healing**.

tive, is the first step to healing. Recognizing that you possess the ability to change your perception, thereby altering old habits of judgment, expectation, and objectivity is a transformational power that realigns you with healthy practices. Destructive patterns of negative thinking, eating dead and depleted foods, living with chronic stress, and staying in unhealthy jobs and relationships have all caused various dis-eases to materialize. Know that every degenerative thought, morsel of dead food, modicum of stress, and denial of true feelings and their withheld expression will take form as dis-ease within the physical body, until you do something to ease it. You can detoxify your strife, producing life with vitality and limitless joy. It all starts with herbs and foods.

Including the two supernatural powers of repairing herbs and boosting foods in your daily routine will give you new awareness, new consciousness, and literally rewire your neural-net to make you more receptive to new ideas, concepts, truths, and creative solutions. The super powers of nature assist in changing the brain chemicals that cause you to stay stuck in thinking habits. Imagine what you could do if you originated every thought that emitted from your brain. Your created thoughts are among the most powerful tools at your disposal to dispel dis-ease and gain ease.

> **Imagine** what you could do if you originated every thought...and if your created thought was among the most **powerful** tool at your disposal to dispel dis-ease.

Use your thoughts, your light powered body, your senses — internal and external — your extra sensory powers, and every resource available to you to heal. DON'T give all your energy to the brain only. Remember its job is to receive information from the senses. Use your whole mind and the rest of your organs that serve an equally important job in the collective operations of how information is processed and formed into your health.

MEET YOUR BODY

"When I let go of what I am, I become what I might be."

LAO TZU

YOUR HEALTH STARTS WITH ENERGY patterns fed into your body, which carries out or materializes those patterns into physical reality. That's a fancy way of saying your physical body does what you tell it to do. Does this mean you consciously tell your digestive organs to metabolize food into usable nutrients? Or tell your lungs to filter air into usable oxygen molecules and pass it along to other body cells? No. But it does mean that with each morsel of food, each passing thought, each unwitting reaction, and each condition to which you subject yourself, you are silently telling your body what to deal with, how you want it dealt with, and are providing the quality of stuff with which to do it. And while you are, perhaps, unconscious of all the "tells" you are communicating, your body responds to all of them according to all the factors involved, and will give you feedback, if you are conscious enough to listen.

> Your physical **body** does what you tell it to do.

WHAT IS YOUR BODY TRYING TO TELL YOU?

Your body loves to communicate with you in every way possible. After all, it exists to serve you and carry out all your choices. It loves to tell you when it is happy, like when you feel warm and fuzzy in your solar plexus (that nerve network around the stomach), and it does its best to tell you when it is struggling, like when your head feels like it may explode. Knowing what our bodies need has fallen by the wayside. As a matter of fact, the thirst mechanism in contemporary people is so weak that 90 percent of the time it is mistaken for hunger. Responding to our body's needs has been de-emphasized over the years until we don't even know what most of the internal organs are called let alone what they do. However, knowing our bodies intimately is the most effective way to be accountable for each of the body's organ functions, health, and happiness.

> Knowing our bodies intimately is the most **effective** way to be accountable for each of the body's organ functions, health, and **happiness**.

When we pay attention and become sensitive to our own body we pick up what is happening on the inside. After healing has taken place, many of the people I have worked with over the years report that they can now feel their spine relax, their ovaries ovulate, their stomach release food into small intestines, bacteria growing in the kidneys, or their heart circulate a happy emotion. Truly knowing your body fills you with a sense of empowerment and confidence that nothing else brings. It becomes exciting when you are so aware of your thinking process that you actually create your thoughts instead of your thoughts creating you.

> It becomes **exciting** when you actually create your thoughts instead of your **thoughts** creating you.

Become more tuned in

to your internal workings by introducing your brain to the various other organs it shares space with. Your brain is but one of the many body parts that serves a specific purpose. Its main job is to gather information from the five material senses and organize it into patterns and sequences that become recognizable and repeatable as a trained response to stimulus. The brain can only act and perform on the information that it has available, and all new information must be patterned into new areas of the brain, literally creating space for incoming intelligence. That is why we often need to see or hear information two to three times before it actually "records" and becomes a retrievable part of us in the memory/sensory bank. It's also why we can hold more information than any computer. We can continually create more memory space.

Every organ in your body performs its function without your brain directing it. Your heart beats, kidneys and liver filter, lungs breathe, cells carry and use nutrients and replicate, and all your systems of digestion, circulation, immunizing, sorting, delivering, and manufacturing function without the benefit of brain command or even awareness. That is why you can form stones, foster infections and even grow tumors without

> You can either train your **brain** to talk to the organs or you can go directly to each **organ** and ask them how they are doing.

your brain becoming involved. Therefore don't depend on your brain for health and wellness information. Your brain can only tell you what it has been told through the material senses. If you have not trained your brain to talk to its fellow organs and systems it cannot advise you. Which means you can either train your brain to talk to the organs or you can go directly to each organ and ask them how they are doing. How is this possible, you say?

Whenever your body has a growing problem it will try to communicate with you via swelling, pressure, pain, rash, gas, odor, redness, itching, acne, obesity, throbbing, bloating, inflexibility, and the various and sundry ways it has to call your attention to a dysfunction. But long before these outward symptoms occur there is an internal upset, imbalance, damage, toxicity, deficiency, or blockage of some sort taking place. You do not need to wait for there to be pain or any other external symptom before you become aware that there is an internal problem brewing.

My ironic sense tells me that the pain mechanism in the human race has developed as a response to ignorance. We have dumbed-down and ignored the internal senses that tell us there is a problem forming. We once had the ability to tell by the taste in our mouth if there were bacteria forming in the stomach or tonsils. We once had the ability to tell of impending infection in the kidneys by the smell of urine. We once had the ability to tell if there were colon impactions forming by the size and color of stool. Since we have ignored these once common senses we have subsequently lost the ability. But there is a way to get them back.

You can perform an organ-by-organ or systems check any time you wish with Body Banter. Checking in with your internal body parts may at first seem impossible, weird, strange, or even crazy. Nevertheless, Jonathan and I developed methods of getting information that have served us well and will serve you too. Your exposure to new information helps you make better choices so that you can be totally accountable for your body's needs, heath, and happiness without relying on or giving your power away.

> New information helps you make **better** choices so that you can be totally accountable for your body's needs, health, and **happiness** without giving your power away.

BODY BANTER - THE SYSTEMS CHECK

Communicating with your body may be a new skill for you, but it is as natural as breathing.

This procedure is best accomplished after reading and understanding the various organs and systems of your body presented in the Systems chapter. When you feel you have a good sense of knowing about how your body works, proceed with this systems check.

In a quiet, tranquil setting, maybe before bed or first thing in the morning, remove any restrictive clothing and shoes, make sure you will not be interrupted, and prepare to relax. Perhaps play some relaxing music, light a colored candle, burn some fragrant incense, or anoint your pulse points with a favorite essential oil. Proceed with relaxing your body in a reclining position, closing your eyes and focusing your intention inward by taking deep breaths, breathing in and releasing, and becoming aware of your heart beats, feeling them become slower and easier as you breathe slowly and deeply. Then clench and relax your fingers, hands, toes and feet, repeating this clenching and relaxing process until you have released all tension in your extremities. Then tighten and relax your shoulders and neck repeatedly until all tension and stress is released. Next, tighten and relax your hips and pelvis repeatedly until all tension is gone, keeping your focus internally on all these tightening and relaxing procedures as they occur.

Now you are ready to talk to your organs individually. Start with the intention of locating and listening to one specific organ, perhaps the one you feel the most drawn to or interested in. Be open to this process and eliminate any possible barriers in your thinking process such as; I don't know how to do this (you will learn as you go) or, I've never done this before (there is a first time for everything) or, I feel uncomfortable doing this (comfort comes with familiarity) or, what if I can't do this (you'll never know until you try) or, what will

I do if I can't do this (you can practice until you are satisfied with your result). Whatever barrier comes up, answer it and eliminate it.

Let's say you have determined it is your heart with which you wish to communicate. Your heart is what pumps emotions into circulation and it loves to circulate positive feelings. Begin a relationship with that organ as you would when meeting another person for the first time. What do you usually do when you meet a new human being? Look them in the eye? Extend your hand in greeting? Decide if you want to get to know them by assessing their form, features, or friendliness? Observe if you are attracted to him or her? Do they have information that is interesting to you? Recall all the ways in which you first encounter another living being and apply the same methods to your own body part, adjusting your methods to fit the appropriate condition or environment. Use your imagination and engage all your senses in the process. How do you imagine your heart looks, what is its texture, how big is it, does it have a smell, what might it feel, how does it work, how does blood flow through it, does it really generate electricity, what happens during its function, does it need something, is there a problem forming? Focus all your energy, thoughts, feelings, and intentions on these inquiries and all these internal dialog questions will be answered by an inner voice or knowing that is inherent and intrinsic to you, coming through or from the organ itself, and floating up to the brain.

At first this process might seem strange, since most of your information has only been received through the five external senses. It may feel like you are just "making it up," or being delusional, but once you have practiced this process you will learn that internal organ information just rises through the tissues, or floats through the circulatory system, or meanders to your mind from beyond normal sensory sources. You will begin to tap into your instincts and intuitions as your various organs share their vast information with the brain, and the brain will learn that it really doesn't know as much as it thought it did.

It takes focus and clarity to accomplish this. If you tend to be easily distracted even by your own thoughts, clear your mind fully before embarking on this conversation.

Listen to what comes. Trust what is exchanged. Begin to relate to and form a bond with this process and the targeted organ. Ask questions and expect answers, wait for them. Be ready to give direction and share information. Anticipate your organ telling you how it heals and what it requires to do so. If it doesn't happen the first time, continue trying and don't give up until you have what you want. Set your standards high and make the decision not to settle for less.

Soon you will begin to find and relate to every part of you until your assorted parts are as familiar to you as any good friend or beloved family member. The organs will become responsive to you, communicative with you, and easy with you as you show interest, give them energy, get to know what they want and need, then provide it for them. You will learn that you can give them direction to repair damage, letting them know that you will supply the herbal tools for them to accomplish the repair. You will understand that each part of you has individual needs, just as the whole of you does, and that you are capable of providing those needs and satisfying every part of you. You may perceive that one organ or system over another needs boosting, and assure it that you will supply the food that boosts its function. You can even inform them of your desired goal and instruct them to help you accomplish it.

Another choice is to go through a series of tests by medical doctors to have them diagnose a problem for you, but remember that they can only tell what's happening to you once symptoms have already occurred and progressed to a critical enough state to show up in their various tests. You, on the other hand, with self-trust and awareness, can determine a developing condition long before symptoms occur (or seek a Raphaology practitioner who can assist you [www.raphaology.info], or take classes in Raphaology to learn more about this process). But, as you can see, the process is so easy to do for yourself.

Body Banter Do's and Don'ts

Do's

- Do take time regularly to check in with your body and do an organ or systems check, connecting and communicating with each part, seeking out developing problems, blockages or overlooked or misinterpreted information.
- Do make a state-of-the-unified-body address to each and every body part on a regular basis, telling it what you would like it to do and what you expect from its performance.
- Do provide all the peak daily nutrients, fluids, sunlight, rest, oxygen, stimulus, exercise, etc., that your body requires.
- Do learn of all the true medicines for your body and their positive herbal effects on the functions of each part of you.
- Do partake of peak foods on a daily basis to provide peak nutrition for peak performance of each organ and system.
- Do apply all of your intuition, awareness, and knowing to the daily practices of peak living and health.

Don'ts

- Do NOT ignore a communication/distress signal, either of a need (i.e. thirst, food, oxygen, sleep) or symptom (i.e. pain, acidity, rash, fatigue) from your body if you want to stay well and well informed.
- Do NOT mask a distress signal by taking a pharmaceutical drug; instead choose an herbal supplement that performs similarly but benefits the problem without toxicity or damage.
- Do NOT put off taking care of the internal environment that promotes or hosts acidity, antibody presence, degeneration, and damage.
- Do NOT accept poor quality or synthetic water, food, air, medicine, or information that will lead to degeneration.
- Love your body as much as it loves you, listen, go inward and communicate. It may help if you know more about your body; its glands, organs, systems, structures, and processes for eliminating toxins.

4 Ways Toxins Leave the Body

"The difference between perseverance and obstinacy is one comes from a strong will, the other from a strong won't."

HENRY WARD BEECHER

EVERY TIME OUR BODY SHIFTS into healing mode it is working to get rid of rancid food build-up or the bacteria that grows on it. We may have been trained to stop this process by thinking that we do not need to suffer the consequences of poor eating habits and therefore reach for a pain reliever, decongestant, anti-acid or the like, but this is effectively stopping the toxins from leaving and creating an intensified and harmful situation.

> Every time our body shifts into **healing** mode it is working to get rid of rancid **food** build-up or the bacteria that grows on it.

In order for healing to take place the toxins must be taken from the body by one or more of the four ways it has to dispose of them:

1. Through the **lungs** by air that you breathe, i.e. coughing, bad breath, and heavy breathing,
2. Through the **skin,** i.e. by fever, sweat, rash, hives, acne, boils, eczemas, and psoriasis,
3. Through the **colon** and sinuses, i.e. in mucous that engulfs toxins and transports them out of the body,
4. Through the **kidneys** and bladder, i.e. through urine and strong uric acids and yeasts.

Dis-ease and its symptoms are merely a product of toxicity in a combination of two basic forms: 1) stored and undigested acidic, rotten, putrefied food has bacteria growing on it and has formed an infection or blockage, 2) toxins emitting from the rotting food and bacteria are not being taken out of the body because the organs have depleted vitamins, fats, minerals, and oxygen and cannot function properly.

> **Dis-ease** and its symptoms are merely a product of **toxicity.**

If the organs of the body do not have access to vitamins, fats, and minerals and are unable to detoxify themselves, then the toxins get trapped in various places in the body where they accumulate, producing a myriad of symptoms.

Every healing process starts with the removal of toxins. Any signs of detoxification can be perceived as a good thing rather than an illness as the body is using its ability to remove stored toxins. Rather than stop or inhibit this process, it can be encouraged, supported, and eased so that energy and health are restored, and the detoxification process is speedy and comfortable.

Our bodies make a fever because elevated temperatures kill bacteria. Fevers can be reduced by drinking thyme tea and taking thyme tea baths, which kills the bacteria so the body can diminish the fever as excess bacteria are diminished. Headaches and stuffy or runny nose can be assisted and foreshortened by lettuce steams or marjoram inhalations and twice daily doses of 1 tablespoon of red wine vinegar or fresh lemon juice added to water, while chest congestion is alleviated with mustard plasters (see remedy section). Nausea is reduced with drops of rosemary essential oil under the tongue and B6 supplementation. Rashes are relieved with topical applications of chamomile tea compresses, extra virgin olive oil, aloe vera gel, and vitamin E oil. The symptoms of healing by detoxification, whether it be headaches, rash, fever, running nose, nausea, behavioral irregularities, etc., are often confused with illness that stemmed from stopping toxins on their way out, or from a toxic build up.

It doesn't matter what the name given to the dis-ease symptom is. What does matter is where the problem originated, which is always from some place in the digestive system. The digestive tract is where healing will start to take place. As we start the healing process, we must first turn to the food we are putting into the digestive tract.

There are two categories of food as far as nutrient absorption is concerned: digestible and indigestible. The foods that are highest in enzymes are the most easily digested and their nutrients readily available, requiring very little bile and therefore minimal stress for the liver where most digestive bile is produced. Foods that are indigestible are low in enzymes, requiring great quantities of bile. They overwork the stomach and liver, often sitting in the small intestines or colon for days, weeks or even years waiting to be digested. During the interim, food nutrients are destroyed, turn rotten, putrefy and then become toxic. Toxic food in the stomach causes burping, acid reflux, heartburn, and ulcer, while food toxins in the small intestines cause allergies, high cholesterol, immune deficiencies, and malnutrition. Other foods make it to the colon for the last phase of digestion but can get stuck there, producing gas and fermentation, which passes through the colon wall, is picked up in the blood stream, and lodges in weak areas of the body causing disease. Colon disorders of this nature may be called irregularity, constipation, irritable bowel syndrome, colitis, ileitis, diverticulitis, etc.

Exacerbating all the digestive system malfunctions are different combinations of STRESS: emotional, physical, and mental. Stress constricts all blood vessels, valves, ducts, lymph nodes and other modes of transporting fluids and oxygen in the body, slowing down the organ function, changing both organ speed and quality of work. Even if a person is in moderately good physical health, stress can cause severe digestive and other functional problems in the body. Stress uses up the vitamin B12 very quickly. Without B12 your body cannot digest food, which then turns into toxins and the disease process has begun.

Exacerbating all the digestive system malfunctions are different combinations of **STRESS**: emotional, physical, and mental.

There are three conduits to healing:

1. **Herbs** stimulate the glands and organs to get rid of toxins and pathogens and to heal organs and tissues by repairing damage.

2. **Vitamins** energize glands into action, supporting production of hormones and restoring organs and tissues to full function.

3. **Minerals** are the bottom line for maintaining the quality of all gland, organs, tissue, bone, and body fluid function with health, energy, longevity, and vitality.

1) The first step is to destroy the bacterial infection or blockage by using antibacterial herbs, and then get toxins moving out by stimulating glands and organs into action through the use of specific herbs for that particular gland or organ (See Color, Organ, Herb Chart Appendix B). Pain and swelling will automatically go away. Antibacterial herbs are: thyme, chamomile, cayenne, horseradish, lavender oil, ABF, and colloidal silver.

RAPHAOLOGY Nature's Antidote for Commercialized Medicine

2) The second step is to restore function to organs with vitamins in order for them to continue releasing toxins and maintain their active working status. The most important vitamins are the B-complex's for digestion and vitamins C, A, E, and D for getting oxygen to cells, restoring organ network support, and assimilating proteins, essential fatty acids, and minerals. These can be attained from raw food or cold-processed food supplements.

3) The third step is to bring digestion to better function so that minerals can be absorbed. Minerals must be returned to the glands and organs to achieve full strength, function, and immunity. The most important minerals are potassium, magnesium, sodium, iron, iodine, calcium, selenium, chromium, and silica.

With these tools available to you, please do not automatically cede your power of self-healing to medical professionals. Pharmaceutical drugs not only mask your symptoms but also prevent you from being aware of the chemical poisoning and organ damage that result.

You can attain health with herbal medicines and maintain perfect health by eating super enzyme foods filled with the peak frequency vitamins and minerals for every gland and organ, and by eliminating stress. The key to reducing stress is to slow down, relax and stop worrying and over analyzing. Remember that all this overworking uses up the reserves of B vitamins, which are the master vitamins to digesting food.

> You can attain health with **herbal** medicines and maintain perfect health by eating super enzyme foods filled with **vitamins** and minerals, and eliminating stress.

BODY SYSTEMS

"Every patient carries his or her own doctor inside."
ALBERT SCHWEITZER 1947

OUR MIRACULOUS BODIES are designed efficiently and will <u>always</u> function maximally and produce health—unless our interference is too great. The self-curing nature of many conditions such as fever, cuts, burns and infection, etc., furnish us with endless examples of how the body tends toward healing. And since the involuntary facilities of the body: breathing, heart beating, fluid exchanging, and digesting all happen without our conscious direction, how can we know what goes on? What makes it all happen?

Our bodies are made up of systems, of which the major ones are comprised of glands and organs. Each system carries out the grand design of the physical body, and is governed by one major hormone producing gland plus a set of organs that use the specific hormones made by the glands. Organ function is fueled by hormones, and glands require light to make hormones. The quality of hormones, and therefore the quality of each system function is dependent on the body's ability to receive light (enzymes, information, energy), manufacture hormones, and deliver them to fuel organ function, support organ, tissue, and nerve groups, circulate and absorb oxygen and nutrients, transport waste, expel pathogens, and exchange fluids. And this all happens without your conscious awareness. Aren't we amazing!

HOW OUR SYSTEMS FUNCTION

If you fell asleep in biology class and can't remember a darn thing about your own body except for what the heart, brain, stomach, and lungs do this will be a review, hopefully more interesting than biology class, creating perhaps a renewed interest on your part because now you are concerned with maximizing your health.

If for years you have been loading your systems with fast or fake food, water substitutes, and pharmaceuticals your systems could be failing. What? My systems could be failing you say! Yes. If you are experiencing headaches, stomach acidity, back aches, acne, lack of energy, smelly poop, stinky sweat, stiff joints, depression, mental fog, or something like any one or more of these symptoms your systems are beginning to fail. Now are you more interested?

> All **health** or dis-ease starts in the digestive system. All dis-ease is based in **malnutrition**, or lack of light.

What causes a system to fail is stored food that has not had the wherewithal to be digested or expelled as waste. All health or dis-ease starts in the digestive system. All disease is based in malnutrition, or lack of light. The body always reaches out for light in all its aspects, and starting with the need for light the body has a set of rules by which it is governed.

One of the body's hard and fast rules is, what it doesn't use or can't get rid of (digestion) it will store (indigestion). This is a good thing if we're talking about storing vitamins, minerals, essential fats, and enzymes. But it's not so good if we're talking about storing artificial coloring and flavoring, synthetic preservatives and drugs, refined or hydrogenated oil, bleached and refined sugar and salt, and enriched conditioned grains. None of these fake foods can be utilized and while some are released as waste, many of these dead foods are stored. Our bodies were never intended to store food,

> One of the **body's** hard and fast rules is, what it doesn't use or can't get rid of (digestion) it will **store** (indigestion).

only its nutrients, and then pass along the fiber as waste.

It's up to us to not only listen to what our bodies are communicating to us, but to also respond by removing the cause of the symptom and repairing whatever damage may have occurred. Preventing or healing dis-ease in an organ saves a system, so pay attention and absorb some knowledge about your body and become wise to its systems.

DIGESTIVE SYSTEM

True health starts with the digestive system, the means by which the body utilizes food; the plant, element, and animal sources of collected light we call enzymes and nutrients. See color insert, illustration 16.1. In the digestive system food is transformed into various energies by the use of enzymes, the energy source for separation and absorption of the different nutrients that the body needs to rebuild, repair, fuel, boost, reproduce, and maintain itself. These are found in our daily foods and fluids. On average, an adult processes two and a half gallons of food, liquid, and digestive secretions daily. It is important to keep the entire digestive tract pH balanced, flora and fauna friendly, free of impaction, well oxygenated, hydrated, highly nutrified, hormonally balanced, and completely functional. Each part of

> **Digestion** means to turn food into liquid. The faster a food can liquefy, the more digestible it is, and the faster its **nutrients** are absorbed.

the digestive system serves a specific and individual function, all of which requires specific and individual herbs and foods to maintain their function.

Digestion means to turn food to liquid so that enzyme and micro-organic factors can act on its individual nutrients. The faster a food can liquefy, the more digestible it is, and the faster its nutrients are absorbed. The digestive process begins each day with the breaking of a nocturnal fast and goes as follows:

1. <u>Carbohydrates</u> from fruits provide the enzymes and energy units that contain and utilize vitamins,
2. <u>Vitamins</u>, which are the impetus for building, scavenging, boosting, eliminating, and restoring provide the basis to make use of proteins,
3. <u>Proteins</u>, which are the building block of cells and tissues in the form of amino acids assist the break down and use of fatty acids,
4. <u>Fatty Acids</u>, which are essential for protection, transportation, and maximizing the application of minerals,
5. <u>Minerals</u>, which is what we are made of, are the basis and bottom line for maintaining the structures and systems of our every body part.

Digestion starts in the eyes, which begin to prepare saliva and gastric juices in the proper amounts and proportions to the anticipated foods, so don't eat while being distracted. Saliva lubricates food being chewed (fifteen times or more is best) and imbeds food with enzymes that begin the assimilation of starches/sugars, the energy units that fuel the food breakdown process. Saliva also kills some bacteria (with immune factors from the tonsils) and disposes of it. Chewing relieves stress and work from the stomach, while tonsil and salivary enzymes protect lower digestive functions from harmful bacteria.

Don't eat while being distracted.

Food then travels down the esophagus (food pipe), past the cardiac valve which closes after food has passed, into the stomach where it is sprayed with hydrochloric acids, which when balanced, ideally acts as a tenderizer and does not burn up nutrients or its own lining. Here food is mixed with pepsin and turned into a soupy mixture called chyme where enzymes can act on carbohydrates, while proteins and fats rely on their own enzymes to be digested.

Ideally, two to six hours after food is mixed with enzymes and acids the pyloric valve at the base of the stomach, releases the liquid food into the duodenum, the first part of the small intestines. As food enters, a signal goes to the pancreas and gall bladder (storage for liver bile) to empty their digestive juices into the duodenum. The duodenum slowly empties chyme into the twenty-seven feet of small intestines where finger like appendages called villi and cilia hairs undulate to move along and assimilate over 80 percent of all foods nutrients, or burn them as heat units known as calories that produce energy for metabolic activity. This is where everything the body needs nutritionally can be released and absorbed into the blood stream directly through the walls of the small intestines, where it is transported directly to the liver.

The liver acts as the filter for any bacteria or toxins that are present on food nutrients that were not taken care of in the mouth, stomach or small intestines. As the main filter for every bite or swallow of food or fluids that enters the body, the liver plays a major role in our digestion and health. It converts cholesterol into digestive bile and stores and uses fatty acids, which are imperative for brain function, immune system function, nutrient and mineral absorption, removal of tissue stored fats, bone marrow production and a host of other life ensuring properties. The liver, our body's main metabolic organ, is also responsible for supervising the distribution of food nutrients, especially fats, to all organ functions as well as containing and eliminating all pharmaceutical, pesticide, and food toxins, so don't let your filter get clogged or disabled.

The liver will do its best to store and neutralize the toxins from non-eliminated waste causing a build up, which stresses and overworks the liver. When the liver is overworked, it will start to degenerate, creating an environment where hepatitis virus can proliferate and active liver cells become replaced by inactive scar tissue, called cirrhosis. An exhausted liver produces abnormal bile that is very sticky and easily forms gallstones in the gall bladder. This abnormal bile cannot effectively digest fats in the smaller intestine, and will either eliminate them totally, causing essential fatty acid deficiency dis-ease, or store the fats in adipose tissue under the skin, causing obesity, or store it in blood vessels causing sticky blood platelets, blood clots, and high serum cholesterol.

Liver bile, which is stored in the gall bladder, is comprised of strong acids and its introduction to the gastrointestinal tract is made through the bile duct. This liver bile, along with pancreatic enzymes, mixes with intestinal flora and fauna to create a pH balance that facilitates the separation and assimilation of individual nutrients through intestinal walls, then on to the liver's filtration where it is marked for delivery by red blood cells, which carry it to its final destination for use in organs, tissues, bones, muscles, teeth, etc.

As discussed earlier, the body's uncompromising rule of storing whatever it cannot use indicates food can be stored for indefinite amounts of time, becoming increasingly more putrid and rotten. Food that is very hard to digest is lacking in enzymes. It requires enormous amounts of digestive enzymes to be manufactured and spends an extensive amount of time waiting for them to be present, if they ever are. Those hard to digest foods include: pork, ham, bacon, cow's milk, cow's cheese, apples, oranges, bell peppers, peanut butter, celery, carrots, white flour, white sugar and white rice, iceberg lettuce, cabbage, grapefruit, and green and yellow onions. Meanwhile, stored food putrefies and releases a large quantity of toxins that off gas and create serious digestive dilemmas. Allergies, Asthma, Candida, and other dis-eases often result from toxins traveling in the blood that get stuck in other parts of the body.

The first attack of these toxins is on the gall bladder/bile duct and the pancreas/pancreatic duct depleting the B-complex vitamins reserve. This is significant because B-vitamins start the digestive process and control the pH balance of digestive acids, raising or lowering digestive stress. Stress reactions will create swelling in the ducts, making the openings very narrow. A repeated occurrence of this can narrow the lengthy ducts down to the point of occlusion allowing almost no digestive juice to pass through. In the event of this, the whole digestive process is severely crippled and food stays in the duodenum even longer, creating toxins that not only put the body out of balance, but starts many dis-ease processes. The weakest part of the body will degenerate more quickly from toxic assaults causing the immune system to work overtime in an attempt to protect the individual from their dangerous effects. If the problem is not corrected, the immune system will falter, causing a number of immune deficiency dis-eases. If the toxins produced have time to creep into the pancreas, then any kind of pancreatic disorder can occur, such as diabetes, hypoglycemia, and pancreatitis.

The pancreas, in addition to being part of the endocrine system, is also the supervisory organ directing digestion from the stomach through to the colon. A sick pancreas slows down the action of the colon, decreasing its efficiency in fluid absorption and eliminating waste. The pancreas is the *main* digestive organ that produces alkalizing bile enzymes, and it uses B-vitamins from which to manufacture them, especially B-12, which neutralizes acidity and initiates the break-down process of food, enabling nutrients to be released and absorbed. If this alkalizing bile is not present the acidic bile continues to break down the food into a heated, rotting, putrefied, toxic mass producing

Stored food putrefies and **releases** a large quantity of toxins and creates serious digestive **dilemmas**.

off gases that will be circulated throughout the body, creating systemic acidity and toxicity, both of which are the perfect host and breeding ground for bacteria, virus, and fungi.

The food fibers and glutens, substances that carry and protect nutrients, are passed on through the long surface area of small intestines. See color insert, illustration 16.2. Fibers clean the walls, villi, and cilia and dispense nutrition as they move along, and then are transferred out through the ileocecal valve and into the colon. As it passes into the first part of the colon, a mixture from the appendix is excreted into the passing substance consisting of friendly bacteria, white blood cells and digestive enzymes that will aid and protect the final process of the food's journey.

Once the mixture of fiber and fluids enters the colon, the residual vitamins and minerals, which are processed along with a host of symbiotic flora and fauna and various yeasts and bacteria perform the job of separating fluid from fiber and mixing fiber with mucous. In this process, 90 percent of all water is removed from fluid digested matter, is passed on to liver and then kidneys, and its volume is compacted, stored (not desirable), or excreted. Large amounts of mucous are made in the walls of the colon both to hold fecal matter together and for protection against harmful bacterial activity. Powerful muscles in the bowel pockets of colon walls contract to facilitate peristaltic action in keeping compacted waste moving toward expulsion. Impactions and harmful growths in and on these bowel pockets form into dis-ease symptoms known as IBS, Crohn's, diverticulitis, polyps, ileitis, cancer, etc.

Any problems that occur along the way of this digestive process are caused from stress, over acidity (pH imbalance), refined and over processed foods, enzyme poor foods, improper flora and fauna, bacterial damage, or essential fatty acid and mineral deficiency. All digestive problems can be overcome with the use of a combination of pro-biotic microbes (found in cultures such as yogurt, kefir, and sour cream), repairing herbs and peak enzyme foods:

Organ	Repairing Herb	Boosting Food
Eyes	Myrrh	Broccoli
Teeth	Lemon Balm	Red onion
Tonsils	Blue Flag	Leeks
Liver	Hawthorn leaf	Crook neck squash
Taste Buds	Red beet	Guava
Pancreas	Thyme	Red kidney beans
Stomach	Centaury	Plum
Small intestine	Centaury	Plum
Colon	Gotu Kola	Red potato
Bile duct	Gotu Kola	Red potato
Gall bladder	Alfalfa	Rasberry
Appendix	Rasberry leaves	Kiwi

Enzymes are the catalyst of every action that occurs in the body. They can be found in the food we eat and are made in the body. Without enzymes the body functions are too slow, nutrition is wasted, dis-ease sets in, and aging speeds up. Always eat foods rich in enzymes (light), vitamins, fats, and minerals (see *Peak Frequency Foods* list, Appendix A).

All suggested foods require only small proportions, i.e. one-quarter cup broccoli, squash, beans, or potato; one-quarter plum or kiwi; two to six raspberries; and one to two teaspoons of red onion or leek. The key is consistency with food: more variety, smaller amounts, with regularity — food as daily medicine.

Enzymes are the catalyst of every action that occurs in the body. Without enzymes **nutrition** is wasted, dis-ease sets in, and aging speeds up.

All suggested herbs are best consumed in extract/liquid form in a glycerin base, for ease of digestion and highest healing concentration. Ten to fifteen drops twice daily with meals is recommended. *Peak Frequency Plant Therapy* offers optimal quality, handmade botanical products with standards far surpassing comparable commercial goods. Visit www.peakherbs.org or www.ifarmacy.com for more information.

HORMONE SYSTEM

The hormone system is made up of seven main endocrine glands that produce organic chemical hormones made from the seven visible colors of the light spectrum. These endocrine glands are known, from top to bottom, as the pituitary and pineal glands, located in the brain; the thyroid gland, located at the base of the throat; the mammary glands, located in the nipples; the kidneys and adrenals, located mid-waist on either side toward the back; the pancreas gland, located above the navel to the left, and the testes and ovaries, otherwise known as the sex glands, located in the groin area. The hormones these glands release are fuel for every organ function, all of which regulate; mental capacity, perceptive abilities, metabolism, respiration, heart rate, circulation, digestion, elimination, fluid exchange, growth rate, sexuality, fear, creativity, etc. See color insert, illustration 16.3.

Hormones are essentially vital and potent for every system of the body. A little bit of hormone goes a long way when considered that if you were to collect all the hormones made by your body over your lifetime they would fit on the head of a pin. The balance of these powerful but delicate organic chemical substances is vitally important. The amount of hormones created and released depends on the body's needs. Levels change in response to stress, blood pressure and gas, digestion demands, immunology, relationships, nutrition, etc.

The **hormone** system functions best when it has abundant supplies of **minerals**, which are available directly from sunlight or found in nutrient and **enzyme** rich foods.

The hormone system functions best when it has abundant supplies of minerals, which are available directly from sunlight or found in nutrient and enzyme rich foods. Brain hormone producing glands need selenium, thyroid needs iodine, mammary glands need iron, kidneys need zinc, pancreas needs chromium, and ovaries and testes need magnesium to maintain their function. When mineral depleted foods are the only choice, high-quality food supplements will provide great quantities of missing elements.

Pituitary

This mind gland, roughly the size of a pea, located in the center brain is known as the master gland. It governs all other hormone-producing glands and manufactures specific hormones that stimulate thyroid, adrenals, testes and ovaries. Pituitary is responsible for our intelligence; memory storage and accessibility; aptitude for receiving new knowledge; formation of our impressions; commanding the creation of thoughts; and having cognition and knowledge. It makes growth hormones that regulate the amount of nutrients taken into the cells, and it secretes feel-good hormones such as *serotonin* and *tryptophan*, along with *melanin*, which affects skin color. It is responsible for receiving information from the five senses and organizing your thinking patterns and cycles. A part of pituitary hormones stimulate the secretion of breast milk and causes uterine contraction for childbirth. Another of its aspects regulates water retention by the kidneys. Pituitary uses the gold color of the light spectrum from which to make its hormones and can be repaired with the herb marigold and boosted by eating lemons.

Pineal

This coneshaped gland in the brain, often referred to as the third eye, is not only the administrator of the body's immune system, it also regulates the biorhythms and aging process. It communicates with and supervises the kidneys and thyroid as the other two main immune regulatory glands, and it is responsible for sexual and menstrual development. Pineal hormones give you the ability to have visual perception through the eyes, to project yourself into the future, and to have clear vision of what you want. It secretes a large number of hormones including *melatonin,* which increases during darkness and allows you to get to sleep, and it inhibits the secretions of *gonadotropins* which accelerates sexual development. Pineal uses yellow light for its hormones, is repaired with the herb mustard and is boosted by eating apricots.

Thyroid

Supervising the metabolic rate of the entire body, the thyroid makes the hormones that the parathyroid distributes for the heat and energy exchange of every body function. Since every single function in the human body, from digestion, to circulation, to thinking, to detoxification, requires metabolism, the thyroid determines the rate at which all processes take place. Its hormones allow you to speak, make decisions, determine what is right for you, and express yourself. Thyroid also produces *calcitonin*, which helps to lower levels of calcium in the blood, caused by eating indigestible calcium in cow's milk or refined salt for instance, that would otherwise build up as calcified hardening in the organs, tissues, and blood vessels. A body overwhelmed with calcification causes the thyroid to stress and lose function. Thyroid supervises the thymus, which produces T-cells (killer immune cells) in its vast network of lymphocytes, and it has the ability to concentrate iodine from foods. Green is the color of light thyroid needs and it is repaired by cayenne pepper and boosted with rosemary.

Mammary

Not generally recognized as significant, nipple hormones are what govern the synchronicity of the highly balanced rhythm between the heart's beating and the lung's breathing; a speed up or slow down in one will cause a responsive balance in the other. Irregular breathing or heart rates affect oxygen absorption, emotional balance, energy levels, mental stability, and motivation. All respiration and lymphatic function comes under tutelage of the mammary glands. Nipple stimulation causes more hormones to be released, which can increase breathing or heart rate, amplify oxygen exchange, inspire motivation, regulate uterine contractions, and boost lymphatic circulation. Blue is the color of light the mammary glands need and it is repaired by American ginseng and boosted by cilantro.

Kidneys/Adrenals

These twins are the main organs to filter all four and a half gallons of blood, lymph and cellular fluids; the kidneys also provide an invaluable service by pH balancing these fluids every minute of the day. The adrenal-kidney complex impacts all the relationship experiences in our lives and manufactures *adrenalin* to give you endurance, body strength and the ability to fight or flee. Stress is managed by the production of anabolic steroids, which stimulate replacement of destroyed cells, while immunity is maintained by the secretion of catabolic hormones, which destroy attacking cells. Another of its hormones is *cortisol* which generates energy, converts carbohydrates into glucose and directs reserves to the liver, while suppressing inflammation. *Aldosterone* regulates the mineral and water balance of the body (electrolytes), keeping blood pressure in check and minimizing dehydration. Kidneys need violet light and are repaired with sarsaparilla herb and boosted with the luscious papaya fruit.

Pancreas

As the organ governing digestion, the pancreas secretes cells that make alkalizing enzymes and B-complex vitamins and, along with liver and small intestines, is responsible for the alkaline side of the pH in the gastrointestinal tract. It makes insulin, which is the glue that binds all nutrients to red blood cells for delivery to organs, bones, tissues, vessels, muscles, teeth, and hair, regulating blood sugar levels and nutritional use. *Glucagon*, a hormone that increases the amount of sugar in blood by causing the breakdown of fats and proteins, is governed by the pancreas, which also manufactures and stores fats and proteins. Because it works to keep all systems of the body in balance, the pancreas is one of the first attack points of stress and needs careful attendance.

While the pancreas is capable of manufacturing copious amounts of B-complex vitamins, if you are a city dweller and are subjected to the unnatural aspects of stress that go with city life, your body cannot produce enough B vitamins to compensate for the stress generated by city conditions and will require the supplementation of B-complex vitamins along with its co-mineral potassium. Pancreas uses orange light from sunshine, needs thyme for repairing and red kidney beans for boosting.

Ovaries and Testes

The ovaries are the twin female hormone producing glands that have a triple function: 1. Making and releasing ovum (eggs) 2. Secreting sexual hormones such as estrogen and the shared hormone between men and women called progesterone. 3. Performing housekeeping services for the entire body. Each twenty-eight days, as stimulated by pituitary gland and regulated by the pineal gland, the ovarian levels of estrogen increase for the purpose of scavenging the body for excess toxins and sweeping them off to the mineral-rich lining of the uterus where they await the monthly waste dump. These hormones are also responsible for puberty, fertility, sexuality, and femininity, as well as the ability to act, endure, create, and reduce fears. When menopause starts, this means hormone levels are dropping and pineal function, which regulates immunity, is reduced.

The testes, located in the scrotum, are the male glands that produce sperm, secrete testosterone and progesterone, and develop sexual maturity to start puberty and determine male potency. Men do not experience menstrual cycles but testicles do perform the same function as ovaries in that they scavenge the body for toxins and sweep them into the mineral-rich prostate where toxins are neutralized. It is important for men to keep their prostate rich in minerals, and not eat mineral stripping foods like watermelon and peanuts. If the testicles cease producing testosterone, the prostate loses its ability to neutralize toxins and becomes susceptible to disease. Repair ovaries and testes with anise, angelica, chaste berry, juniper berry, noni, and yellow pansy, while boosting with foods such as chocolate, corn, fenugreek leaves, mango, pear, and whole wheat.

Hormone Gland	Repairing Formula	Hormone Booster Formula
Pituitary	Mind-Inyan	Pituitary
Pineal	Focus-Chapi	Pineal
Thyroid	Self-Identity-Chanli	Thyroid
Mammary	Motivation-Wagle Shun	Mammary
Kidneys/Adrenals	Relations-Yumeni	Kidneys/Adrenals
Pancreas	Balance-Wi	Pancreas
Ovaries/testes	Peace-Luta	Hutahlex

Please note the introduction of two types of liquid herbal formulas from *Peak Frequency Plant Therapy* (www.peakherbs. org) that work specifically with each of the seven hormone glands: Repairing Formulas and Hormone Booster Formulas. These indicate the types of Peak Frequency Plant Therapy extracts that apply specifically to **Repairing** hormone glands, i.e.

- Pituitary gland is repaired by *Mind-Inyan* Formula and **Boosting** hormone glands, i.e.
- Pituitary gland is boosted with *Pituitary* Hormone Booster Formula.

Common dosage is ten to fifteen drops twice daily with breakfast and dinner.

COMMUNICATION SYSTEM

The brain, heart, hormones, cells, and nerves together form the communication system of the human body. See color insert, illustration 16.4. This system is responsible for processing, relaying, accessing, and storing information, thinking, directing movements and actions, emoting, perceiving pain, sleeping, temperature, immunity, and more. This is the vital link between our internal world and external events and conditions. The sensory organs and cells of the nervous system receive external information and relay it to the brain, which in turn sorts, prioritizes, and organizes instantaneously and passes it on to the organs, tissues, and cells so that they may adapt and change as necessary. Internally, the heart, fluids, and blood elements circulate emotional/energy factors that are communicated either to the brain axis or the involuntary impulses of solar plexus, kidneys, etc. The intra-network of relay information goes through and is initiated by the individual cells themselves. Each cell has its own brain and these cell brains are in constant communication and directives with each other.

The nervous system works electrochemically, fueled by the electrical stimulus made by the heart. Tiny impulses, or currents, are generated through millisecond exchanges of charged potassium and sodium particles across nerve cell membranes and then pass along the nerve fibers without causing any change to its physical appearance. This system has two main parts: central and peripheral. The central part consists of the brain, heart, and spinal cord, and the peripheral part consists of the wire-like nerve network throughout the body. It is composed of over 36 billion neurons, or nerve cells, that receive and transmit messages by means of electrical and energetic impulse. When the impulse from the brain arrives at the end, called the effector, activity is then stimulated. When information from single cell brains is transmitted to nerves, involuntary reactions are stimulated. See color insert, illustration 16.5.

The brain has three main parts: the cerebrum, cerebellum, and brain stem. The cerebrum receives information, "thinks" about it, processes it, and sends it on to related areas. The cerebellum balances and coordinates function. The brain stem connects the cerebrum to the spinal chord and through the thought process regulates respiration, heart rate, eye movement and pupil dilation or contraction, and neck and head movement.

The brain receives two main types of messages from the nerves: relaxing, or contracting. These influence whether to act or react, fight or flee, feel stress or calm. The heart both generates electricity and receives nerve and cell impulses of electrical and energetic information. Both the brain and the heart are cognitive parts of the communication system, assisted by the "little brain" in each of our body cells. The brain is able to receive and relay information from external sources and the heart is able to transmit information to the brain from internal sources.

The part of the brain concerned with emotions and memory response is called the limbic system. It is the area through which all sensory information coming up through the spinal cord enters the brain, and through which all motor commands flow back downward. It is also the center through which information from all the special sense organs of the cranium enters the brain. The limbic system, or emotional brain, has the densest collection of neuropeptide bonding sites in the brain. The limbic system is where chemical information from its neurons and from the blood (matter) connects with electrical nerve impulses in the brain (thought) and where the true union between mind, energy, and matter takes place.

The little known function of this part of the brain includes the *amygdala, cingulate gyrus, hippocampus,* and the *hypothalamus.* It is these areas that are especially concerned with emotions that deal with neuropeptides, a secondary nervous system. Differing from the synapses that send, pass, and receive

BODY SYSTEMS

ical stimulus from neuron to neuron, neuropeptides have
tion on individual cells, carrying "feelings" generated
thoughts or by emotional conditions. Hence, it is not
surprising that emotional stress or overload can lead to
psychological and physical illness.

There is no state of mind that is not mimicked by the state
of the immune system. Every repressed emotion is stored in the
body cells, the unconscious body, by means of neuropeptides,
and memories are stored in neuropeptide receivers. The
language of emotion is intrinsically capable of generating
every kind of self-awareness and creating opportunities for
self-healing.

Peptides are embedded in the membranes or outer covering
of neurons and all other cells, and are attracted and collected
with receptor sites on cell membranes; there can be many on
each cell. The binding of an information molecule (*ligand*) to a
receptor site is like a key fitting into a keyhole. Scientists now
believe that only 2 percent of communication with the brain
occurs via synapses and 98 percent by information molecules
such as hormones and neuropeptides, which act over longer
distances.

Dr. Candace Pert, author of *Molecules of Emotion*,
observed that spontaneous healing happens when destructive
emotions are released, and conversely, dis-ease happens as
a result of anchoring destructive emotions in the thinking
process. This phenomenon of the body's ability to produce
"molecules of emotion" can generate the feelings of anger,
love, hope, or depression almost instantaneously by the
production of billions of neuropeptides that circulate in
fluids and lock into billions of cells causing every cell to
experience the same "feeling" at the same time from the top
of the head to the soles of the feet. When we get red in
the face, or sweat all over, this is not caused by messages
from the brain but are rather produced at the cellular level
when neuropeptides bind to receptors. These peptides can
produce mental, physical, and emotional states individually

or simultaneously. Just a thought can provoke a chemical change for every cell. Can you imagine what a clear and persistent inner vision of health, abundance and happiness would do to your body?

Each cells membrane consists of microtubules that provide the cytoskeleton or scaffolding of the cell. These microtubules are perfect hexagonal lattices that display incredible intelligence and organizational abilities; serving as circulation, transporting of materials, internal motion, processing and communicating information, organizing neighboring cells into unified motion, regulating synaptic connections, and releasing neurotransmitters.

Just as insults and shocks, stress and depression are communicated and imprinted on every cell, the reversal of these cellular imprints can be achieved with *somatid* pulsations that literally shed light bodies on cells by participating in feelings of joy, love, inspiration, compassion, and positive excitement that generate peptides to provoke positive changes in thinking and action. Emotional expression is tied to a specific flow of peptides and therefore either disturbances or balances in psychosomatic and immuno-support/suppress functions.

A daily supply of high-enzyme, nutrient rich foods to the body provides the nerves, peptides and cell membranes with peak resources for accurate transmissions, which reduces our daily stress and increases our daily health with every tool in the box. Daily frustration, worry, mental over-load, limitations, obligations, shame, and constraints can be more harmful to nerves than big trauma. Prolonged emotional stress can lead to nerves breaking down every bit as much as stressed thinking breaks down immunity and digestion.

We can be proactive by balancing work with relaxation, hurrying with slowing down, seriousness with laughter, and inactivity with dancing, exercise, frolicking, a little wild-and-craziness, and taking accountability for our health by replacing dis-ease with ease.

Element	Protects	Boosted with
Vitamin E	Nerves	Magnesium (whole wheat, figs, or almonds)
Horseradish	Spinal Cord	Passion Fruit
Chamomile	Brain	Avocado
Vitamin C	Arteries	Raspberries
Yerba Santa	Heart	Mandarin Orange
Positive thoughts	Cells	Self-Trust

IMMUNE SYSTEM

We are all familiar with the five main senses, but our sixth sense, the immune system, is one we need to become more familiar with in order to peak-up and maintain our health. The immune system is a highly sophisticated group of organs, glands, ducts, nodes, hormones and structures that is comprised of the pineal gland, the tonsils, adenoids, thymus, spleen, bone marrow, appendix, adrenals, and the network of lymph nodes that transport white blood cells throughout the body. See color insert, illustration 16.6. Our defense system recognizes the individual antibodies, attackers, mutagens, parasites, bacteria, virus, and fungi that even the brain can't identify, and converts that recognition into activating the indubitable immune response.

The cycle of antibodies, parasites, and toxins in the human body is a constant and "normal" occurrence as their potentially destructive presence is daily disposed of by a healthy immune system. Lymphocytes, leukocytes, macrophages, phagocytes and a host of other "killer" immune cells are the marshaled forces that constantly patrol the entire body. When an anti-body predator is detected, each of these "killer" cells are immediately put on alert with up-to-date information and go into action to find and remove the unwanted visitor. A full inventory of predatory antibodies is kept in the memory banks of each type of "patrol" cell and is called upon to recognize and remove or destroy every form of destructive entity and activity. When a new predator is recognized, the updated

Illustration 7.1

Raphaology Light Chart

Location of Light Centers on the Physical Body

Light from the sun enters the body at the top of the head and ideally flows through the body and out the feet. As our bodies receive light, which is information energy in waves, we process it using all our experiences and abilities, including our genetics. If light does not get stuck or trapped somewhere along its path, its healing energy flows through us into SKA (our earth) and becomes available to every living inhabitant.

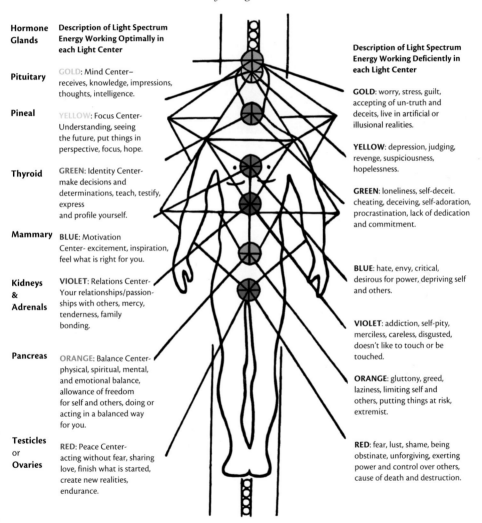

Hormone Glands

Description of Light Spectrum Energy Working Optimally in each Light Center

Pituitary

GOLD: Mind Center– receives, knowledge, impressions, thoughts, intelligence.

Pineal

YELLOW: Focus Center- Understanding, seeing the future, put things in perspective, focus, hope.

Thyroid

GREEN: Identity Center- make decisions and determinations, teach, testify, express and profile yourself.

Mammary

BLUE: Motivation Center- excitement, inspiration, feel what is right for you.

Kidneys & Adrenals

VIOLET: Relations Center- Your relationships/passion-ships with others, mercy, tenderness, family bonding.

Pancreas

ORANGE: Balance Center- physical, spiritual, mental, and emotional balance, allowance of freedom for self and others, doing or acting in a balanced way for you.

Testicles or Ovaries

RED: Peace Center- acting without fear, sharing love, finish what is started, create new realities, endurance.

Description of Light Spectrum Energy Working Deficiently in each Light Center

GOLD: worry, stress, guilt, accepting of un-truth and deceits, live in artificial or illusional realities.

YELLOW: depression, judging, revenge, suspiciousness, hopelessness.

GREEN: loneliness, self-deceit. cheating, deceiving, self-adoration, procrastination, lack of dedication and commitment.

BLUE: hate, envy, critical, desirous for power, depriving self and others.

VIOLET: addiction, self-pity, merciless, careless, disgusted, doesn't like to touch or be touched.

ORANGE: gluttony, greed, laziness, limiting self and others, putting things at risk, extremist.

RED: fear, lust, shame, being obstinate, unforgiving, exerting power and control over others, cause of death and destruction.

As each frequency band of light has a visual color on the spectrum, it possesses other aspects in addition to color, such as tone or sound, shape or symbolic dimension, smell or odor, vibrational wave patterns or texture, emotional feelings, and a host of aspects that cannot be experienced by the senses of the physical body. These realms are experienced in the psyche, super-conscious, spiritual, or metaphysical bodies.

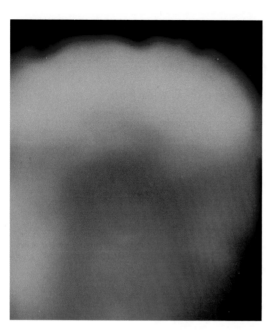

Illustration 8.1: Kirlian Photography isolates radiant energy, known as the Meisner Field, emitted by the human body in spectrums of light. The healthier you are the more colorful and dense the light field becomes.

Illustration 16.1: Digestive System is where total body health is attained or disease prevails. Here food is transformed into various energies by the use of enzymes: the higher food's enzyme content the more energy and vitality digestion produces.

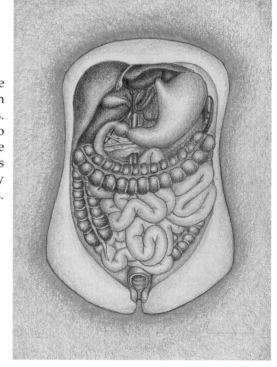

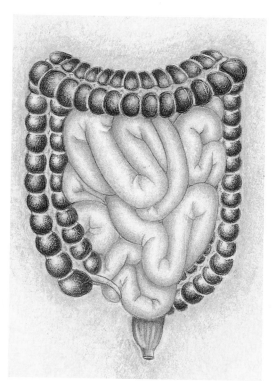

Illustration 16.2: Gastrointestinal tract provides the passage of nutrients and fluids through its walls using villi, bile, enzymes, peristalsis, and a host of micro-flora that create the conditions for foods to nourish, ferment, or compact.

Illustration 16.3: Hormone System is made up of the seven main hormone glands, taking their resource material from the seven main colors of sunlight to produce hormones. From top to bottom: Pituitary, Pineal, Thyroid, Mammary, Kidney/ Adrenal, Pancreas, and testes or ovaries.

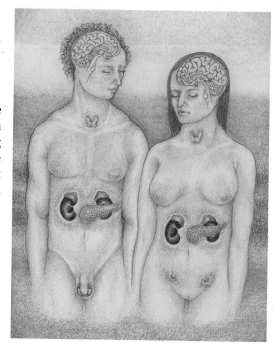

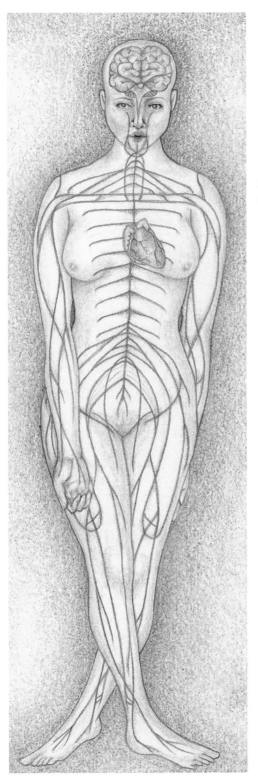

Illustration 16.4: Communication System, comprised of brain, heart, cell membranes, and nerves convey all information throughout the body, and provide a vital link from the internal to the external environment.

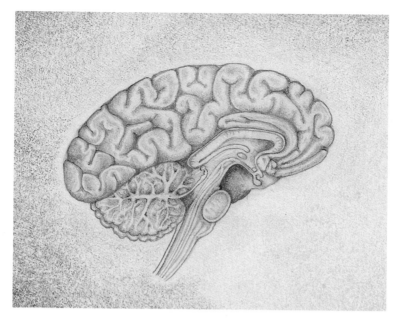

Illustration 16.5 : Brain matter has three main parts; cerebrum, cerebellum, and brain stem that all receive, send, and direct messaging through nerves and can formulate thought with imagination.

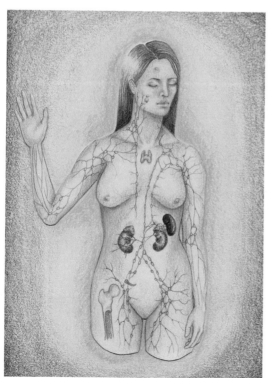

Illustration 16.6: Immune System serves to identify, scavenge and eliminate pathogens, debris, acidity, mutagens, and parasites, while providing a sophisticated network of healthy activity in all areas of the body.

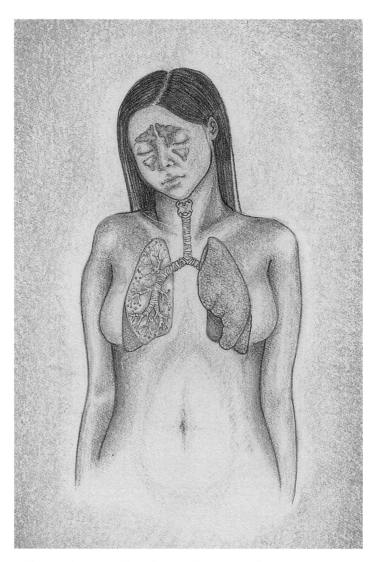

Illustration 16.7: Respiratory System exchanges oxygen and fluids with gasses and toxins via nose and mouth. Capable of exchanging 2 -4 cups of fluids daily, lungs deliver oxygen molecules to every body cell and expel toxins with every breath.

Illustration 16.8: Bronchia extend into bronchioles with round nodules called alveoli situated at each ending that expand and contract to create surface tension through which oxygen molecules pass to red blood cells.

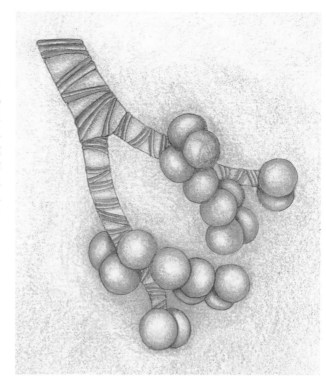

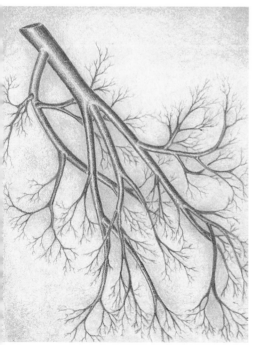

Illustration 16.9: Rib muscles contract to expand lungs, allowing intake of air to go through a tree-like branching of bronchi with each breath. It directs oxygen down to the smallest stem throughout the lungs.

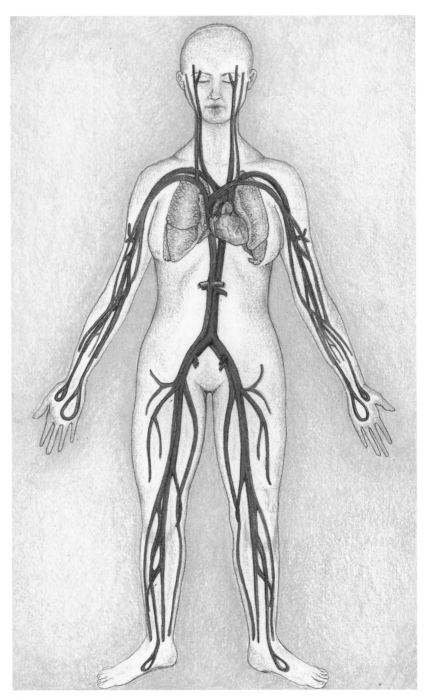

Illustration 16.10: Circulatory System transports every life supporting element through fluid constituents that deliver oxygen, nutrients, and hormones, and expel gasses, toxins, and pathogens. Blood fluids comprise roughly 2 gallons that travel through arteries, veins, capillaries, and ducts.

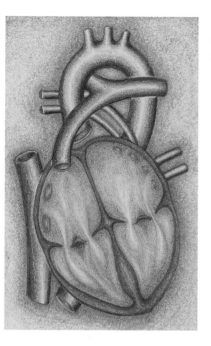

Illustration 16.11: Heart muscles contract causing a vortex action that spins blood and emotions throughout the body.

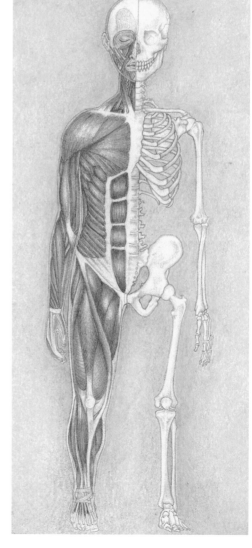

Illustration 16.12: Structural System is framed by bones, muscles, tendons, ligaments, and connective tissue providing the framework for every body movement. Comprising a mineral mass of over 206 bones, our structure never stops rebuilding to achieve strength and flexibility.

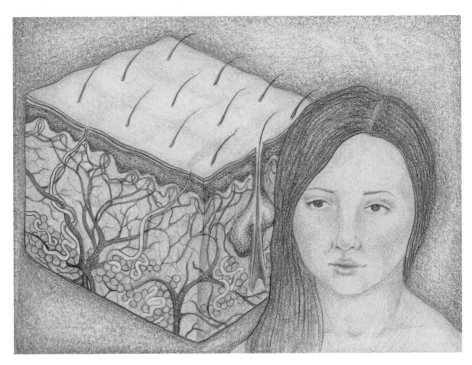

Illustration 16.13: Skin, hair, and nails are our protective barriers and provide a visual indication of inner health. Skin is the largest organ, hair is the antenna for the liver, and nails protect sensitive fingers and act as tools.

Illustration 16.14: Nails show dramatic changes in their shape, texture, color, and growth signaling changes of internal conditions that precipitate occurrences such as arthritis, diabetes, or Candida, all of which are mineral deficiencies.

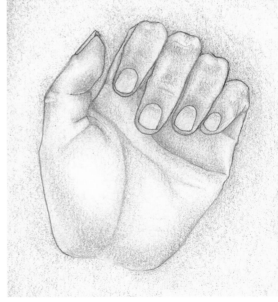

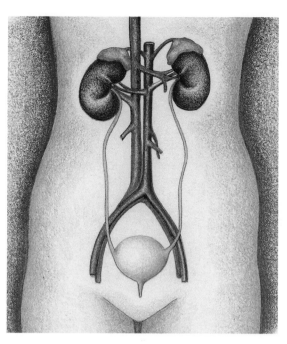

Illustration 16.15: Urinary System transports fluid waste consisting of uric acid and other fluids from kidneys and adrenals after careful filtration, rendering urine through ureter tubes to bladder and out the urethra.

Illustration 16.16: Female Reproduction, consisting of ovaries, fallopian tubes, uterus, cervix, and vagina, and produces hormones, stem cells, and ovum is stimulated through mind and heart functions. They are all internally located and provide the criteria necessary for perpetuating the human race.

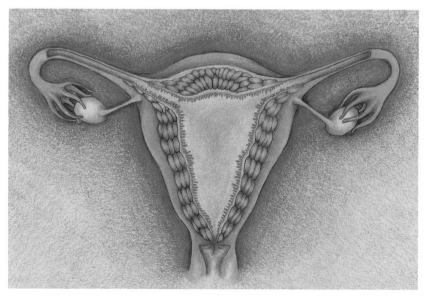

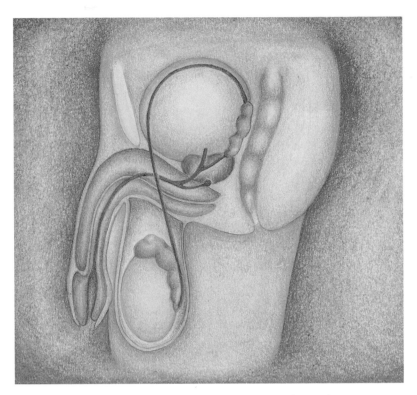

Illustration 16.17: Male Reproduction consists of testicles, prostate, Cowper's gland, penis and scrotum and produces hormones, sperm, seminal fluid, and stem cells. Ejaculation occurs to deliver sperm swimming in seminal fluid to fertilize the females ovum resulting in conception.

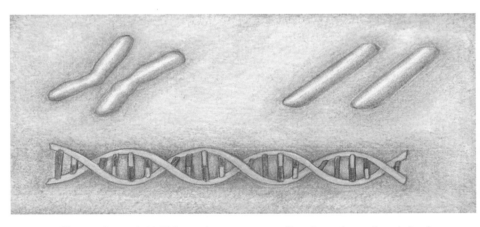

Illustration 16.18: Above is a conceptualization of man's original chromosomes on the right, and on the left is the degenerated shape of what are considered "normal" chromosomes today, and the genetic material, DNA, that is contained within them.

have dumbed-down knowledge of what's good for you, not okay to suppress your innate healing abilities with drugs, nor to give away your accountability for healing to professionals, then your quiver is now full of arrows that can shoot holes in the commonly accepted substandards of healthful living, and hit the bull's-eye on the target of your higher choices.

We learned that we are our own healers and that nature provides the true

> We are our own healers and **nature** provides the true medicine.

medicine. With the knowledge of plants and foods as our reparative and daily medicines, you can make new choices and actually take accountability for true health and well-being. By taking to heart this revolutionary information about healing that works with the natural synergy of your body, you can customize it for your particular and unique set of parameters. In doing so you will gain and maintain the standards of living that you want. But you are required to do the

> You are **required** to do the work.

work. Even though new things may seem difficult at first, as with everything else, it gets easier with each attempt, until you find that you have actually created ease, rather than dis-ease.

Our changing understanding of biology and health will help us navigate this turbulent period in our planet's history. How each of us actively participates in this global evolutionary shift has already exceeded the quest for answers, shifted past decisions, and moved into the action of our choices. Along with the new information contained in this book comes fresh realizations of your potential as a co-creator of our collective reality. You are in command of your immediate reality: what you create and manifest with your thoughts, food, expressions, relationships, and actions. You remain the most powerful individual when it comes to your body's health, happiness, and purpose. You are part of the most potent experience of universal proportions. You help pilot the course that determines the future of us all. You cannot fail when you determine and stand in your own truth.

Getting You Started

*"Not a shred of evidence exists in favor
of the idea that life is serious."*

BRENDAN GILL

SO NOW YOU ARE INSPIRED. You've decided you want to be healthy, but all this new stuff seems pretty overwhelming. Take a deep breath and just relax. You're fine. You can do this. Many others have and reaped untold rewards. You deserve this.

Starting at the ground floor, go into the kitchen, and take a discerning look. Begin by opening your pantry, spice cupboard, pots and pans cabinets, refrigerator, storage container shelves, silver and serving ware drawers, and plastic wrap, aluminum foil and baggie trays. We're going to take inventory first, then get rid of everything that's toxic. Let's do this right!

Replacing everything at once can be expensive, exhausting, and time-consuming, so start with what's doable first, and continue as you are able. Make mental, or actual, notes so that you can prioritize and adjust for your pocketbook, schedule, energy, and availability.

THE 20 MOST IMPORTANT THINGS TO TAKE OUT OF, AND PUT INTO YOUR HOME

What to Take Out

Get rid of, throw away, remove, 86, adios, trash, and round file any of the following:

From the Kitchen Counter top:
1. Microwave oven

From the Herb and Spice Cabinet:
1. All table salt, even if it's kosher or sea salt
2. Black and white pepper
3. Garlic and onion powder
4. Seasoning salts with MSG or table salt (if it's not Real Salt™ it's trash)
5. Coffee creamers and artificial flavors

From the Cupboards:
1. Plastic and wooden cutting boards (they grow bacteria and spread it to your food, no matter how well you clean them).
2. Aluminum cookware; pots, pans, cookie sheets (it's okay to keep those if you are willing to line them with unbleached parchment paper for baking), wok, serving trays, bread and pie pans, and casserole dishes
3. Anything with a non-stick coating (it off-gasses into your food)
4. Plastic ware: food storage containers, glasses, bowls, and dishes

From the Refrigerator:
1. Anything in the line of "I can't believe it's not butter" substitutes or margarine
2. Cow's milk anything: cheese, ice cream, cottage or cream cheese

3. Mayonnaise or Miracle (that you're still alive) Whip or ketchup

From the Pantry:
1. Canola oil, and peanut, walnut, and vegetable oils, lard, or shortening
2. Refined, bleached, enriched, self-rising flour
3. White sugar and artificial sugars
4. South American, decaf, or instant coffee
5. White rice, oat meal, or rye bread or cereal

From Under the Sink:
1. Any product with rubbing alcohol, or isopropyl alcohol
2. Anything with ammonia or chlorine bleach

From the Bathroom:
1. Toothpaste with fluoride
2. Deodorant/antiperspirant with aluminum chlorhydrate

What to Put In

Stock the Counter Top with:
1. Toaster oven (it takes less space, doesn't cause free radicals, and cooks in about the same time)

Stock the Herb and Spice Cabinet with:
1. Real Salt™
2. Cayenne (red) pepper
3. Elephant garlic and red onion powder
4. Real Salt™ Seasoning (see recipe, appendix D)
5. Replace powdered or artificial creamers with organic heavy whipping cream, or goat, almond, or rice milk

Stock the Cupboards with:
1. Glass or marble/granite cutting boards (even though they are porous they don't sponsor bacterial growth)

2. Stainless steel, glass, ceramic, copper, or cast iron cookware
3. Well-seasoned cast iron pans are non-stick if you heat them first and use a light coating of sunflower oil (you can put oil in spray bottle to apply)
4. Glass storage containers (it's okay to have plastic lids, just place wax or parchment paper between food and lid)
5. Stainless steel, copper, ceramic, or silver serving ware

Stock the Refrigerator with:
1. Organic, unsalted butter or goat butter
2. Goat or sheep milk and their cheeses, ice cream, cream cheese
3. Sandwich spreads made from grape seed oil or organic tofu, or make your own (see recipe appendix E)
4. Duck eggs to replace chicken eggs

Stock the Pantry with:
1. Extra virgin olive oil, grape seed, and hemp oils for salads, and cold pressed sunflower, safflower, sesame, and coconut oils for cooking
2. Whole grain wheat, barley, whole wheat pastry flours are rich in minerals, or brown rice flour is gluten free and alkalizing
3. Sucanat™ (natural sugar cane), raw honey, grade B maple syrup, date or coconut sugar, or unrefined corn fructose
4. Papua New Guinea coffee, the only alkalizing coffee
5. Brown rice, rolled barley meal, and non-bleached/un-enriched whole grain breads or cereals

Stock Under the Sink with:
1. Natural alcohol cleansers and witch hazel astringent are far more effective and do not harm skin and attract parasites
2. Herb-based disinfectants and food-grade hydrogen peroxide do a better job without the loss of brain and sinus cells

Stock the Bathroom with:
1. Fluoride-free toothpaste: propylus and myrrh work better to protect teeth from cavities without harming the kidneys
2. Aluminum-free deodorant: mineral sticks are a natural deodorizer and don't stop lymph circulation

THE MOST IMPORTANT DO'S AND DON'TS OF FOOD

What Foods to Avoid

Apples

Black tea, green tea, iced tea

Bell peppers; green, red, and yellow

Brown potatoes (Russet), Yukon, or white

Cabbage, bok choy, Brussels sprouts

Carrots

Celery

Coffee, South American

Cow milk products (cheese, milk, ice cream)

Eggs (chicken)

Regular garlic

Grapefruit

Ham and pork products , especially bacon

Hot peppers

Iceberg lettuce, red leaf, and romaine lettuces

NutraSweet, Aspartame

Oats

Oranges

Peanuts, walnuts, pecans, hazelnuts

Pepper (black and white)

Shark

Soda pop, especially cola drinks

Squash

Sugar and salt (refined)

Tuna

Watermelon
White flour
White rice
Yellow and white onions
Processed, enriched, FD&C foods
Chemically preserved foods

See Appendix A: *Peak Frequency Food List* for the total list of super enzyme, high nutrient foods in all their categories and have fun!

Excellent Protein Sources
Almonds
Almond milk
Avocado
Beans: Anasazi
   Red kidney
   Soy (organic only)
   White (navy, cannellini, lima)
Bison/buffalo meat
Duck eggs
Feta cheese (sheep or goat milk)
Goat milk, cheese, yogurt
Grains (esp. wheat and wheat sprouts)
Mushrooms
Red lentils
Red potatoes
Rice milk (organic)
Romano cheese (sheep milk)
Salmon (wild caught)
Sprouts: alfalfa, wheat, sunflower, broccoli, red clover
Soy milk (organic only)
Tofu (organic only)
Trout (wild caught)
Whole wheat pasta

Excellent Essential Fatty Acid Sources

The human body cannot digest minerals without fatty acids.

Almonds
Almond milk
Avocado
Cashews
Feta cheese (goat or sheep milk)
Goat; milk, cheese, yogurt
Grains, (barley, buckwheat, rice, wheat)
Oils: cold, expeller pressed, and extra virgin
      Avocado oil
      Flaxseed oil
      Grape seed oil
      Olive oil (Mediterranean region)
      Safflower oil
      Sunflower oil
      Wheat germ oil
Olives
Pecorino romano, manchego (sheep milk cheeses)
Pine nuts
Soy milk (organic only)
Sunflower seeds

21 Day Peak Frequency Food Challenge

"What may be done at any time will be done at no time. There is no time like the present."

SCOTTISH PROVERB

THIS IS A CHALLENGE, no, an opportunity, for you to really feel the difference in what eating high-quality foods can do to boost your energy, your thinking, your digestion, circulation, sexuality, creativity, and vitality. Even if you think you're eating well now, even if you feel pretty good about how and what you eat and drink, and even if you don't believe a word of anything you read, you can take this challenge and risk being amazed at what a delightful benefit just changing your daily foods can bring.

You will be truly flabbergasted at the taste sensation of eating foods that feed your body, mind, and emotions. You will realize that you were formerly feeding your taste buds, your persuasions, or eating for convenience. But now you will comprehend that there really is such a thing as soul food. You will be left with no doubt that real food tastes

> There is food that truly sustains **life**, maintains health, and offers you untold benefits.

really good. You will know that there is food that truly sustains life, maintains health, and offers you untold benefits.

Once you have eaten only *Peak Frequency Foods* for twenty-one days, go back to your old eating habits. You may just find that the gourmet junk you used to eat doesn't taste so good any more. The smell of rotisserie chicken's rancid fat may turn your stomach. The salt on your favorite French fries will now taste acidic and make you thirsty and retain water. The ranch dressing on iceberg lettuce salad that used to satisfy your taste will now taste like chemicals. The artificially sweetened drink you used to love will now burn your tongue and give you a headache.

Your body will now be able to recognize the difference between a fake food and a peak food and become far more discerning. You will taste the difference between refined salt and Real Salt™, between refined sugar and real Sucanat™, between rancid fat and a fatty acid. And be prepared that you won't like the fake stuff anymore. Your body may even reject the fake stuff after having been provided the real deal, and possibly punish you for giving it death-on-a-platter.

ACCEPTING THE CHALLENGE

When you are ready to start, go to appendix A for the full list of Peak Frequency Foods and get your kitchen prepared. Use up, discard, or give away all the old foods, stock up your new foods, and set the date for your big adventure. Meanwhile, here are a few tips on eating the peak way. You can ensure proper digestion and absorption of full nutrition with these simple measures:

- Let each meal consist of 60 percent raw, fresh food, and 40 percent cooked food.
- Use more beans/legumes and grains together to make a complete protein rather than having animal proteins several times per week.
- Before eating, take a moment to really look at your food so that all your digestive organs can properly prepare the correct saliva, bile, and enzymes.

- Chew your food thoroughly, fifteen to thirty chews per bite.
- Never eat under stress, on the run, or in a hurry, take your time.
- Never eat while doing something else, such as driving a car, reading a book, or watching TV.
- Always use B-complex vitamins and potassium to reduce digestive stress and help the pancreas produce alkalizing bile enzymes.
- Use the spices of thyme, cayenne, turmeric, and cloves in your cooking.
- Avoid processed, prepackaged, and convenience foods that are hard to digest, especially those with canola or palm oil, artificial preservatives, and poor quality salt.
- Avoid hydrogenated and partially hydrogenated fats and oils, such as margarine, shortening, and purified oils.
- Resist soda and sports drinks, instead drinking 8 glasses of pure, clean water each day.
- And last, but not least, be appreciative, grateful and enthusiastic about the food you eat.

Okay. Get started on your new life by putting this plan into action. Know that every good thing has been provided for you by our earth mother, and that the answers to all your healing needs are readily available. You are a loved and important part of all that is and have the power to do any and every thing you want.

APPENDIX A

Peak Frequency Foods

We know that our cars need fuel to run. The better quality of fuel we put into them, the better gas mileage they get, the better they run. Put a poor quality fuel or oil into them, and the engine clogs and begins to run poorly and soon all the systems are negatively affected. Why is it that we recognize and respect the relationship between the health of our automobiles and the fuel we choose for them while we often overlook that same relationship between our bodies and fuel we provide for them?

Peak Frequency Foods are the optimal fuel for our system. They are the foods that contain the highest amounts of enzymes, nutrients, and life force factors, and are the most sustaining for the human body as daily medicine. Foods are the daily nutrition that constitutes the fuel for life, and herbs are the repairing factors that comprise the tools to heal, detoxify, and regain function. Once healing has taken place, maintaining health is accomplished with daily maintenance of foods. Not all so-called foods accomplish this purpose. Some things that we routinely consume are degenerative, dis-easing, and destructive. They are not included on the *Peak Frequency Foods* list.

Please take the twenty-one-day challenge and eat only foods from this list for three weeks so that you can feel the difference in your energy, clarity, and vitality that takes place with just a change in daily foods.

RAPHAOLOGY *Nature's Antidote for Commercialized Medicine*

BERRIES

Bilberries
Blackberries
Boysenberries
Cranberries
Gooseberries
Hawthorn berries
Juniper berries
Loganberries
Mulberries
Raspberries
Red currants
Shizandra berries
Strawberries

VEGETABLES

Artichoke
Asparagus
Arugala
Avocado
Beets (red)
Broccoli
Caper
Cauliflower
Crook neck squash (yellow)
Cucumber
Eggplant
Fennel
Green beans
Horseradish
Jicama
Leek
Lettuce, butter, endive,
   spring mix, radiccio
Kale
Mushroom-chanterelle, rei
   shi, cremini,
porcini, shitake
Mustard greens

Olives
Red onion
Red potato
Spinach
Swiss chard
Tomato (roma, plum, heir-
   loom)
Watercress
Yams

FRUITS

Apricots
Banana (after five hours of sun)
Cantaloupe
Cherry
Coconut
Date
Fig
Grape (red, blue, black)
Guava
Honeydew melon
Kiwi
Lemon/Lime
Mango
Mandarin orange
Nectarine
Papaya
Passion fruit
Peach
Pear
Persimmon
Pineapple
Plum
Pomegranate
Prune
Star Fruit
Tangerine

SPROUTS
- Alfalfa sprouts
- Bean (mung) sprouts
- Broccoli sprouts
- Buckwheat sprouts
- Fenugreek sprouts
- Mustard sprouts
- Red clover sprouts
- Wheat sprouts
- Sunflower sprouts

GRAINS
- Amaranth
- Barley
- Buckwheat
- Corn
- Kamut
- Millet
- Rice-(brown) basmati, california, wild
- Wheat

BEANS
- Anasazi beans
- Kidney beans (dark red)
- Lima beans
- Red lentils
- Soy beans, edamame
- White beans (navy, cannellini, white kidney)

HERBS/SPICES
- Allspice
- Anise
- Bay leaf
- Basil
- Cardamom
- Cayenne
- Chives
- Cilantro
- Cinnamon
- Cloves
- Cumin
- Dill
- Elephant garlic
- Fenugreek
- Ginger
- Hawthorne leaves
- Marjoram
- Morinda/Noni
- Mustard (seed/leaves)
- Nutmeg
- Oregano
- Paprika
- Peppermint
- Rosemary
- Sage
- Spearmint
- Tarragon
- Thyme
- Turmeric
- Vanilla bean
- Yucca

NUTS/SEEDS
- Almond
- Anise seed
- Brazil nut
- Caraway seed
- Cashew
- Fennel seed
- Flax seed
- Hemp seed
- Pine nut
- Sesame seed
- Sunflower seed

MEATS/FISH wild caught
  Orange roughy
  Buffalo/Bison meat
  Jumbo shrimp
  Salmon
  Lake trout

OILS-extra virgin, first cold pressed,
expeller pressed
  Avocado oil
  Corn oil
  Flaxseed oil
  Grape Seed oil
  Olive oil, extra virgin
    (mediterranean region)
  Safflower oil
    (best for frying)
  Sesame oil
  Soy oil (organic)
  Sunflower oil

NATURAL SWEETENERS
  Brown rice syrup
  Date sugar
  Fructose (unrefined from
    organic corn)
  Honey (raw or unfiltered)
  Maple syrup (grade B)
  Molasses
  Sucanat ™(sugar cane
    natural)

MILK PRODUCTS
  Almond milk
  Butter (unsalted)
  Buffalo/Bison milk and cheese
  Coconut milk
  Goat milk, cheese, yogurt
  Rice milk
  Sheep cheese, feta,
    manchego
  Sour cream (daisy or
    wallaby brand)
  Soy milk or cream
  Whipping cream, heavy,
    organic

MISCELLANEOUS
  Baking powder
    (Rumford brand)
  Beer (Coors Light)
  Braggs Liquid Amino's™
  Brewer's yeast
  Carob
  Chocolate (dark)
  Coffee (Papua New Guinea)
  Duck eggs
  Honey comb/royal jelly
  Morinda /Noni juice
  Nutritional yeast (KAL)
  Bee pollen, propylis, royal jelly
  Vinegar (red wine, brown rice, bal-
samic)
  Wine, red (aged 7 yrs. or more)

For more information about Raphaology and Peak Frequency
Foods, visit www.raphaology.info. See you there!

How To Read the Chart:

The **Color** column represents the color of light in the spectrum of frequencies from which glands in the human body make their hormones.

The **Gland/Organ** column represents the specific systems consisting of hormone producing glands and their corresponding life support organs that use the spectrum of light in its field for healing.

The **Herb** column represents the single herb that contains the specific property for repairing the gland or organ directly in line across from the listed body part.

The **Food** column represents the one food that boosts the function of the corresponding body part directly across the line.

As light enters the physical body through the pituitary gland, the master hormone supervisor, and separates out into the spectrum of colors, each one passes down the matrix of light/hormone centers to furnish each gland and system organ with the energy to perform its peak function.

This differs even from the common practice of treating symptoms that originate from an organ by viewing health from a holistic perspective, taking into consideration that the hormone producing glands furnish hormones that fuel each organ function. This is important because if hormones are out of balance, the corresponding organs become dysfunctional. Treating organs alone without going to the causal gland/hormone is insufficient. Healing takes place with the all-encompassing combinations of herbs and foods.

Color	Gland & Organ	Herbs	Foods
Mind Gold	**Pituitary Gland** Gallbladder Large & Small Brains Spleen Teeth, Sinuses Tonsils	Marigold (Calendula) Alfalfa Chamomile Witch Hazel Lemon Balm (Melissa) Blue Flag	Lemon Raspberry Avocado Grapes (red, blue, purple) Red Onion Leeks
Focus Yellow	**Pineal Gland** Inner Ear Liver Bones	Mustard Suma Leaves Hawthorne Leaves Marshmallow	Apricot Ginger Crook Neck Squash Barley
Self Identity Green	**Thyroid** Eyes, Olfactory Taste Buds Spinal Cord Nerves	Cayenne (Capsicum) Myrrh Red Beet Horseradish	Rosemary Broccoli Guava Passion Fruit
Motivation Blue	**Nipples** Heart, Lungs Respiratory Tract Lymph	American Ginseng Yerba Santa Cranberry Golden Rod	Cilantro Mandarin Orange Figs Bananas (after 5hrs in sun)
Relations Violet	**Kidneys & Adrenals** Bladder Skin Solar Plexus	Sarsaparilla Kava-Kava White Willow Bark Passion Flower	Papaya Tomatoes/Roma Pineapple Hawthorne Berry
Balance Orange	**Pancreas** Appendix, white cells Colon, Bile duct Stomach, Small Intestine, Pancreas duct	Thyme Raspberry Leaves Gotu Kola Centaury	Kidney Beans (red) Kiwi Red Potatoes Plums
Peace Red	**Testicles, Ovaries**	Anise Seed Noni (Morinda) Juniper Berry Angelica Rt. (Dong Quoi) Chaste Berry Yellow Pansy	Mango Wheat Corn Pear Fenugreek Chocolate (cacao bean)

Real Salt™ Seasoning Blends

Real Salt is unrefined sea salt mined from ancient dried sea beds in Redmond, Utah.

General Seasoning Blend

Keep this on hand to sprinkle on vegetables, salads, eggs, or anything you like.

1 tablespoon Real Salt™
1 tablespoon dry mustard
1 tablespoon elephant garlic powder
2 teaspoons dried marjoram
2 teaspoons dried dill weed
2 teaspoons red onion powder
2 teaspoons dried basil
2 teaspoons dried thyme
1 teaspoon dried lemon peel
Dash cayenne

Vegetable Blend

Use this blend in stir-fries with a bit of lemon juice or on any vegetables.

1 ½ tablespoons red onion powder
1 ½ tablespoons toasted sesame seeds
1 tablespoon dried chives
1 tablespoon dried tarragon
1 tablespoon dry mustard
1 ½ teaspoons dried dill weed
1 tablespoon Real Salt™
Dash cayenne

Seafood Blend

Try this on poached, grilled or baked fish, either before or after cooking.

1 tablespoon dried dill weed
1 tablespoon dried thyme

1 tablespoon dried fennel
1 tablespoon dried sage
1 tablespoon dried marjoram
½ tablespoon ground bay leaf
1 ½ teaspoons dried chives
1 ½ teaspoons red onion powder
1 ½ teaspoons Real Salt™
Dash cayenne

Italian Blend

Try this for salads, Italian sauces, or handmade Italian breads and pizza sauce.

1 tablespoon dried rosemary
1 tablespoon dried marjoram
1 tablespoon dried oregano
1 tablespoon dried basil
1 tablespoon dried elephant garlic powder
½ teaspoon anise (if you like licorice flavor)
1 ½ teaspoons dried cilantro
1 teaspoon dried thyme
½ tablespoons Real Salt™
Dash cayenne

Mexican Blend

This is great for enchilada sauce, rice seasoning, tacos, and sour cream dip spicing.

1 tablespoon red onion powder
1 tablespoon elephant garlic powder
2 tablespoons cumin powder
2 tablespoons paprika powder
1 tablespoon coriander powder
2 tablespoons dried cilantro
2 tablespoons dried and ground lemon peel
1 teaspoon Anaheim chili powder
⅛ teaspoon cayenne pepper
2 tablespoons Real Salt™

Spicy Blend

For those who like a lot of flavor with a little kick.

1 tablespoon elephant garlic powder

1 tablespoon red onion powder

1 tablespoon dried and ground lemon peel

1 tablespoon dry mustard

1 tablespoon dried and powdered horseradish

1 teaspoon allspice

1 teaspoon coriander

1 teaspoon marjoram

½ teaspoon low-medium heat cayenne pepper

1 tablespoon Real Salt™

APPENDIX D

**Homemade Mayonnaise and Ketchup
with Salad Dressing Bonus**

For more recipes and food tips visit www.raphaology.info.

Mayonnaise - yields 1 cup
> 2 ounce organic soft tofu
> 2 tablespoons fresh squeezed lemon juice
> ½ cup extra virgin olive oil
> ¼ to 1 teaspoon dry mustard (to taste)
> ¾ teaspoon Real Salt™

Combine tofu, lemon juice, ¼ cup oil, dry mustard, and Real Salt in food processor or electric blender. Cover and blend at low speed until well mixed. Increase to high and remove cover to add remaining oil in a thin, slow, steady stream until all oil and mayo is smooth and creamy. Store in glass container and keep refrigerated and use within 10-14 days.

Raw Ketchup - yields 1 quart
> 2 cups Roma tomato sauce:
> 1. Blanch 9-12 Roma tomatoes (dip in boiling water for 3-4 minutes, run under cold water to stop heat, then slip skins off)
> 2. Cut open tomatoes, then remove seeds with spoon
> 3. Purée tomato solids in food processor or blender
>
> Add into food processor: 1 cup sun-dried Roma tomatoes
> ⅓ cup raw honey
> ¼ cup grade B maple syrup
> 6 fresh basil leaves or 1 tsp. dried
> 6 pitted dates
> ½ teaspoon allspice
> 1 tablespoon paprika
> 1 tablespoon tamari
> 2 teaspoons elephant garlic powder or 1½ tablespoons pressed elephant garlic

¼ cup red wine vinegar

dash to ¼ teaspoon cayenne (to taste)

dash to ½ teaspoon Real Salt™ (to taste)

Store in covered glass jar in the refrigerator for up to 2 months.

Fresh Salad Dressings

Fat Burner Dressing

6 tablespoons extra virgin olive oil

1 teaspoon balsamic vinegar

2 teaspoons fresh squeezed lemon or lime juice

1 teaspoon red wine vinegar

1 tablespoon <u>Kal</u> nutritional yeast

1 teaspoon <u>Bragg</u> liquid amino's

½ teaspoon Real Salt™

½ teaspoon dried sweet basil herb

½ teaspoon thyme

Dash elephant garlic powder

Dash red onion powder

Dash cayenne

Italian Anti-Acid Dressing

4 tablespoons extra virgin olive oil

1 tablespoon balsamic vinegar

1 tablespoon red wine vinegar

1 teaspoon raw honey

¼ teaspoon oregano

½ teaspoon marjoram

¼ teaspoon sweet basil

¼ teaspoon Real Salt™

¼ teaspoon elephant garlic powder

Honey Mustard Dressing

4 tablespoons extra virgin olive oil

1½ tablespoons prepared mustard

1 ½ tablespoons raw honey
1 tablespoon fresh lemon juice
¼ teaspoon Real Salt™
Option: ½ teaspoon dried dill

French Fat Burner Dressing

4 tablespoons extra virgin olive oil
1 tablespoons red wine vinegar
1 teaspoon lemon juice
½ teaspoon prepared mustard
½ teaspoon raw honey
¼ teaspoon Real Salt™
½ teaspoon sweet basil
¼ teaspoon thyme
Dash cayenne

These dressings can be made fresh for a salad to serve four people or for a single serving salad, refrigerating the rest. These recipes can also be made in four to ten times the quantity and kept in the refrigerator. When doing so, add ½ teaspoon liquid lecithin to emulsify the ingredients and keep oil from separating and getting solid.

APPENDIX E

For more information on the single herbs and combination formulas of <u>Peak Frequency Plant Therapy</u> please visit www. peakherbs.org

NATURAL REMEDIES FOR COMMON AILMENTS
Cross Reference

Absent-mindedness: gotu kola, American ginseng, mind, pituitary, ginko biloba

Acne: sarsaparilla, echinacea, colloidal silver, ABF, B-complex

ADD/ADHD: B-complex, kava-kava, passion flower, lavender essential oil (topical)

Adrenal exhaustion: sarsaparilla, American ginseng, relations, kidneys/adrenals

AIDS: myrrh, red clover, AVF, noni, B–complex, food grade hydrogen peroxide

Alcoholism/drug addiction: cayenne, grass-C, goldenseal

Allergies: chamomile, nettles-iron & calcium, sarsaparilla, B-complex, bee propylis, bee pollen, royal jelly

Anemia: nettles-iron & calcium, alfalfa, American ginseng, circulation Improving

Anti-acids: chamomile, centaury, horsetail, alfalfa, barley essence

Anti-clotting: rice-E, thyroid, white willow bark

Anti-depressant: kava-kava, passion flower, thyroid, focus

Anti-inflammatory: chamomile, horsetail, juniper berry, sarsaparilla, alfalfa

Anti-histamine: sarsaparilla, nettles-iron & calcium, grass-C, bee pollen or propylis

Anxiety: kava-kava, passion flower, B-complex, SFF, kelp-iodine, noni

Appendicitis: red raspberry, sarsaparilla, chamomile, goat milk

Arrhythmias: hawthorn leaf and berry, yerba santa, heart harmony, motivation, mammary

Arthritis: alfalfa, juniper berry, slippery elm, horsetail, Joint support

Asthma: gotu kola, peppermint, yerba santa, chamomile, breathe easier, alfalfa, golden rod, lobelia, ABF, TNF

Athlete's foot: colloidal silver, juniper berry, tea tree oil

Back/muscle ache: B-complex, muscle relaxing, white willow, SFF, horseradish, mustard plaster (topical)

Bad breath: centaury, sarsaparilla, balance, B-complex, ginger, thyme, peppermint

Bedsores: juniper berry, horsetail, colloidal silver, colloidal gold, circulation improving, white willow

Bladder dis-ease: passion flower, cranberry, sarsaparilla, ABF, relations, colloidal silver

Bleeding: cayenne, kelp-iodine, American ginseng

Blood poisoning: sarsaparilla, cayenne, colloidal silver, sage, TNF, thyme, grass-C

Blood pressure: sarsaparilla, hawthorn berry, real salt, grass-C, B-complex, SFF, (for reducing) and cayenne (for elevating)

Blood thinner: white willow (instead of aspirin)

Bone density: nettles-iron & calcium, marshmallow, red clover, alfalfa, B-complex

Breast milk increase: blessed thistle, marshmallow, marigold, B-complex

Breast milk arrest: sage

Bronchitis: American ginseng, blue flag, yerba santa, sarsaparilla, AVF, B-complex, breathe easier

Bruises: witch hazel, marigold, B-complex, grass-C, white willow, rice-E

Burns: chamomile, aloe vera (topical), raw honey (topical)

Cancer: AVF, ABF, noni, American ginseng, red clover, red beet, tea tree oil, apricot kernel oil, anti-parasite therapy, FG hydrogen peroxide

Candida: myrrh, AFF, brewer's yeast, ABF, centaury, chamomile, colloidal silver, anise, goldenseal

Canker sores: B-complex, centaury, chamomile, red wine vinegar, FG hydrogen peroxide, baking soda (topically)

Childbirth: red raspberry, ginger, passion flower

Cholesterol lowering: hawthorn leaf, alfalfa, barley essence, dandelion root tea, grass-C

Chronic fatigue: American ginseng, sarsaparilla, AVF, B-complex, kelp-iodine

Circulation (poor): grass-C, sarsaparilla, circulation improving, ginger, peppermint

Colic: peppermint, chamomile, wild yam, anise

Colitis: centaury, sarsaparilla, balance, ABF, AVF, B–complex

Common cold: ABF, AVF, thyme, echinacea, sage, marjoram, cayenne, B-complex

Conception/infertility: peace, hutalhex, B-complex, American ginseng, angelica, cayenne, gotu-kola, noni, juniper berry

Constipation: alfalfa, thyme, red potato water, chamomile, anise, psyllium husk

Convulsions: American ginseng, gotu kola, marigold, colloidal gold

Coronary heart dis-ease: American ginseng, heart harmony, hawthorn berry, B-complex, yerba santa, grass-C

Coughing: blue flag, anise, raw honey, chamomile, AVF, B-complex

Dental problems: myrrh, colloidal silver, ABF, lemon balm

Depression: self-identity, focus, mustard, noni, passion flower, kava-kava, thyroid, pineal

Diabetes: balance, thyme, glucose adjusting, nettles-iron & calcium, American ginseng, goldenseal, cinnamon, chromium

Diarrhea: thyme, sarsaparilla, TNF, ABF, B-complex, wheat-magnesium, golden seal, raw red potatoes

Dizziness: American ginseng, gotu kola, circulation improving, suma, horsetail, mind, passion

Dry skin: rice-E, yam-A plus D, olive oil, white willow, B-complex, sarsaparilla

Ear infection: tea tree oil (around ear topically), suma, ABF, garlic ear pack

Energy increase: American ginseng, B-complex, noni, thyroid, balance, kidneys/adrenals

Eczema: American ginseng, white willow, yam-A plus D, relations, kidneys/adrenals

Fear: angelica, anise, fenugreek with thyme, peace, American ginseng, juniper berry, noni

Fever: thyme, B-complex, chamomile, sarsaparilla, ABF, colloidal silver

Gall stones: alfalfa, nettles-iron & calcium, dandelion root tea

Gangrene: alfalfa, sarsaparilla, chamomile, circulation improving, cayenne, plus tea tree oil and colloidal copper (topically applied)

Gastritis: anise, sarsaparilla, centaury, balance, B-complex, slippery elm

Gonorrhea: sarsaparilla, ABF, AVF, relations, American ginseng, lemon balm

Gout: chamomile, sarsaparilla, horsetail, juniper berry, ABF, B-complex, cranberry, alfalfa, circulation improving, grass-C

Hangover: American ginseng, thyme, cayenne

Headache: chamomile, ginger, peppermint, horsetail, TNF, circulation improving, B-complex, red wine vinegar

Heart Problems: wheat-magnesium, yerba santa, heart harmony, red raspberry leaf, CoQ10,

Heartburn: centaury, ginger, peppermint, anise, sarsaparilla, TNF, balance, B-complex, baking soda in water, red wine vinegar in water, food grade hydrogen peroxide

Hemorrhoids: witch hazel, inside of banana peel (topical), B-complex

Herpes/fever blister: lemon balm, l-lysine, AVF, colloidal silver, B-complex, chamomile, FG hydrogen peroxide, red wine vinegar

Hives: sarsaparilla, goldenseal, nettles-iron & calcium, chamomile, plus colloidal silver and lavender oil (both topically applied)

Hot flashes: chaste berry, peace, hutalhex, juniper berry, evening primrose oil, black cohosh, noni

HRT (hormone replacement therapy): angelica, chaste berry, noni, wild yam root

Immune dis-ease: echinacea, motivation, focus, relations, pineal, mustard, kidneys/adrenals, American ginseng, caraway seed

Indigestion: peppermint, anise, centaury, chamomile, ginger, B-complex, colloidal silver, food grade hydrogen peroxide

Infections: ABF, sarsaparilla, chamomile, thyme, echinacea, colloidal silver (bacterial), colloidal gold (viral)

Inflammation: chamomile, ginger, cayenne, sarsaparilla, AVF, balance, self-identity, colloidal silver

Infertility: peace, hutalhex, angelica, B-complex, SFF, mind, pituitary, relations, juniper berry

Influenza: thyme, chamomile, ABF, sarsaparilla, echinacea, B-complex, colloidal silver, alfalfa, horsetail

Insect bite: sarsaparilla, raw honey, TNF, chamomile, plus topical applications of tea tree oil and FG hydrogen peroxide (diluted)

Insomnia: passion flower, chamomile, mustard, ABF, balance, focus, mind, self identity, thyroid, hops, sleep deeper

Irritable bowels: centaury, gotu kola, anise, balance, B-complex, ABF, colloidal silver, slippery elm, SFF

Joint problems: slippery elm, joint support, horsetail, juniper berry, silica

Kidneys dis-ease: relations, kidneys/adrenals, sarsaparilla, cranberry, SFF, chamomile, American ginseng, colloidal silver

Kidney stones: cranberry, dandelion root tea, nettles-iron & calcium, kidneys/adrenals

Kidney infection: sarsaparilla, ABF, silver, TNF, chamomile, cranberry, B-complex, horsetail, kidneys/adrenals

Liver dis-ease: hawthorn leaf, American ginseng, chamomile, colloidal silver, ABF, e.v. olive oil, red raspberry leaf, alfalfa

Memory loss: mind, gotu kola, pituitary, cayenne, perception, marigold, chamomile, ginko biloba, B-complex, memory reviving

Menstrual problems: angelica, suma, noni, chaste berry, SFF, mind, pineal, peace, hutalhex

Menopausal problems: chaste berry, peace, angelica, juniper berry, evening primrose oil, black cohosh

Migraines: chamomile, peppermint, gotu kola, circulation improving, mind, SFF, horsetail, juniper berry, marigold, pituitary

Morning sickness: B–complex (B6), ginger, red raspberry, nettles-iron & calcium, red clover, ginger, peppermint

Motion sickness: B–complex, thyroid, ginger, peppermint, balance, pineal

Muscle inflammation: witch hazel, muscle relaxing, horsetail, chamomile, B-complex, amino acid complex, lactase, L-lysine

Nail problems: horsetail, alfalfa, nettles-iron & calcium, B-complex, super minerals, silica, plus topical applications of tea tree oil and olive oil

Nausea: ginger, B-complex, ABF, AVF, American ginseng, peppermint, colloidal silver

Nervousness: alfalfa, chamomile, AFF, American ginseng, noni, kava-kava, B-complex, SFF, rice-E, passion

Obesity: weight loss, gotu kola, B-complex, ABF, relations, kidneys/adrenals, balance, thyme, letting go, restoring

Osteoarthritis: alfalfa, nettles-iron & calcium, super minerals, B-complex, red clover, joint support, centaury, marshmallow, wheat-magnesium

Pain: American ginseng, white willow, ABF, AVF, APDF, juniper berry, B-complex, chamomile, thyme, grass-C

Pancreas dis-ease: thyme, balance, pancreas, B-complex, cayenne, chamomile, gotu kola, blackstrap molasses

PMS: angelica, suma, peace, mind, focus, letting go, B-complex, hutalhex

Prostatitis: peace, angelica, noni, juniper berry, hutalhex, chamomile, B-complex, super minerals

Psoriasis: ABF, ABV, B-complex, yam-A plus D, hawthorn leaf, sarsaparilla, relations, kidneys/adrenals, white willow, B-complex

Rash: chamomile, sarsaparilla, white willow, B-complex, Yam-A plus D, alfalfa

Sleep disorders: hops, sleep deeper, passion flower, SFF, mind, pituitary, gotu kola, chamomile, thyroid, kidneys/adrenals, wheat-magnesium, L-theonine

STD (sexually transmitted disease): sarsaparilla, lemon balm, peace, hutalhex, ABF, AVF, juniper berry, colloidal silver and sgold, B-complex

Snake bite: sarsaparilla, TNF, B-complex, plus topical applications of lavender and tea tree oils (all repeated with frequent applications)

Sore throat: blue flag, ABF, AVF, B-complex, Real Salt™ gargle, chamomile

Stool softener: thyme, psyllium husk, gotu kola, red raspberry leaf

Stomach problems: centaury, peppermint, ginger, cayenne, colloidal silver, FG hydrogen peroxide

Stress: SFF, kava-kava, passion flower, mind, focus, pituitary, relations, B-complex

Tetanus: juniper berry, sarsaparilla, chamomile, white willow, ABF, AVF, colloidal silver

Thrush: myrrh, ABF, AFF, colloidal silver

Thyroid dis-ease: cayenne, thyroid, self-identity, B-complex, rosemary essential oil

Toothache/abscess: myrrh, tea tree oil, B-complex, colloidal silver

Toxic shock: TNF, B-complex, sarsaparilla

Tumor arrest: red beet, AVF, FG hydrogen peroxide

Ulcer: centaury, gotu kola, cayenne, anise, red wine vinegar, B-complex, balance, chamomile, papua new guinea coffee

Urinary tract infection: sarsaparilla, ABF, silver, thyme, relations, cranberry

Vertigo: American ginseng, horsetail, circulation improving, mind

Vision: focus, lemon balm, myrrh, mustard, pineal

Warts: juniper berry, myrrh, AVF, gold, sarsaparilla, cranberry, dandelion root tea, anti-parasite therapy, latex from dandelion (topical)

Whooping cough: blue flag, anise, sarsaparilla, tea tree oil (topical)

Wounds: thyme, lemon balm, golden rod, B-complex, marshmallow, sarsaparilla, grass-C, slippery elm bark

Wrinkles: horsetail, focus, pineal, grass-C, B-complex, Amino acid complex, L-lysine, silica

Yeast infection: myrrh, sarsaparilla, horseradish, horsetail, AFF, brewer's yeast

Should any symptoms persist, please consult the services of a professional health care provider. None of the above information has been reviewed or approved by the FDA and is not intended to diagnose, prescribe, treat, or cure disease. All contained material is offered with the intent to educate, inform, and support self-healing.

APPENDIX E

AFTERWORD

As a Professor and Doctor of Raphaology Medicine, I am not a medical doctor nor do I practice medicine as taught in medical schools. My training has come from the examples, teachings, and practices of my late beloved husband, Jonathan: Thunder: Wolf and from our visits and sharing know-how with the many Healers and Osages of the indigenous Oriental, native Red Men, Inkan, Viking, and Egyptian worlds.

Jonathan's and my experiences have come from life lessons and their practicality, using this invaluable knowledge in healing ourselves and honorably teaching and assisting thousands of others on their self-healing path. We learned that there is no magic pill; each of us can only exercise our ability to heal ourselves.

Our education, though not formal, stems from our own healing paths and the revealing inter-relationships we participated in with aboriginal people, plants, animals, and elements that are filled with universal truths and are abundantly offered by Creation for our health. Our authority to teach healing precepts is derived from private experiences as well as those we've shared with thousands of individuals who hold a scope of information far surpassing the conventions and curriculums derived from public books. A modicum of that information is put forth in this body of work, offered with the highest intent to benefit our fellow humanity and our cherished planet, who is our mother.

The educational format of information compiled from the wealth of Jonathan's and my experiences can be obtained through the Universal College of Indigenous Medicine encompassing the College of Raphaology Medicine.

You are invited to participate at www.raphaology.info.

INDEX

absent-mindedness, 178

accountability
> decision to heal, 151–154
> for dis-ease, 9–10, 54, 55, 69–70, 72, 74, 103, 142

acid reflux, 81

acne, 178

ACTH, 26

ADD/ADHD, 178

adenoids
> repairing herbs/boosting foods, 108
> role of, 106, 107, 109

adrenal exhaustion, 178

adrenalin, 26, 97, 125

adrenals
> location of, 17, 97
> repairing/boosting herb formulas, 99
> repairing herbs/boosting foods, 97, 108, 126, 171
> role of, 97, 106
> stress hormones and, 26, 97, 125
> in urinary system, 124, 125
> violet light and, 17, 97

adrenocorticotropin, 26

AIDS, 178

alcoholism/drug addiction, 178

aldosterone, 97

allergies, 4, 81, 90–91, 178

ampulla, 128

amygdala, 101–102

anabolic steroids, 97

anemia, 123, 178

animals, 148–149

anti-acids, 178

antibiotics, 57–59

antibodies, 104

bathroom

    adding items to, 159

    removing items from, 157

B-Complex Vitamins

    benefits of, 62–63, 64–65, 83–84, 112

    digestive system and, 91–92

    dosages, 63

    stress and, 82, 98

bedsores, 179

bile, 81, 89, 90, 91–92

bile duct

    repairing herbs/boosting foods, 93, 171

    role of, 90–91

Biology of Belief, The (Lipton), 139

bladder

    in detoxification process, 80

    repairing herbs/boosting foods, 126, 171

    in urinary system, 124, 125, 132

bladder dis-ease, 179

bleeding, 179

blood poisoning, 179

blood pressure, 124, 179

blood thinner, 179

blood type diets, 59

blood vessels

    repairing herbs/boosting foods, 114

    role of, 111–112, 113

blue light, mammary glands and, 17, 97

body, 71–78

    Body Banter, 74, 75–78

    communicating with, 72–78

    healing symptoms. *See* healing symptoms

    introducing brain to organs, 72–74

    medical tests for, 38, 77

Body Banter, 75–78

    do's and don'ts, 78

nature of, 74
procedures for, 75–77
body systems, 85–139. *See also* organs
Body Banter and, 74, 75–78
circulatory system, 110–114
communication system, 100–104
digestive system, 87–94
functioning of, 86–87
genetic system, 133–139
hair, 122–123
hormone system, 94–99
immune system, 104–108
nails, 123–124
reproductive system, 17, 127–133
respiratory system, 109–110
skin, 120–122
structural system, 115–120
symptoms of failure, 86
urinary system, 124–126
bone density, 119, 179
bone marrow
repairing herbs/boosting foods, 108
role of, 105, 115
bones, 115, 116–120
conditions, 115, 117–120
repairing herbs/boosting foods, 108, 119, 171
brain, 101–103
in Body Banter, 74, 75–78
cell brains, 100, 101
components of, 101
heart and, 7, 76
herbs and, 34
hormone producing glands, 95
introducing to other organs, 72–74
messages received from nerves, 101
and Raphaology medicine, 6–7

repairing herbs/boosting foods, 104, 171
role of, 6–7, 73
breast milk arrest, 179
breast milk increase, 179
breathing, 96–97, 109, 148. *See also* respiratory system
bronchitis, 179
bruises, 179
burns, 179
burping, 81
bursae, 116

caffeine, 24, 69
calcification, 96
calcitonin, 96
calcium, 117–119
food sources, 119
supplements, 118
calories, 89
cancellous bone, 115
cancer, 179
cure rates, 66
natural cancer elimination, 52, 66
Rife Ray Machine and, 48
spontaneous remissions/recoveries from, 42–43
war on, 52
candida, 90–91, 179
canker sores, 179
capillaries, 112
carbohydrates, 22, 24
in digestive process, 88, 89
carbon dioxide, 109–110
Carlin, George, 25
catabolic hormones, 97
cells
brains of, 100, 101
components of, 103

colloidal copper, 137

colon

in detoxification process, 80, 81–82

repairing herbs/boosting foods, 93, 108, 171

role of, 92, 105–106

colon dis-ease, 81–82, 92

colors

auric spectrum, 20–22, 30

foods and, 35

frequency spectrums of, 27

hormone glands and, 16–17

mineral light and, 22–24

Raphaology Chart, 170–171

Color Therapy, 12

commercial medicine, 33, 45–47. *See also* pharmaceuticals

cancer cure rates, 66

doses of nutrients and, 65

tools of, 3, 41

common cold, 66, 180

communication system, 100–104

brain, 101–103

heart, 100, 101

nervous system, 100

repairing herbs/boosting foods, 104

conception/infertility, 180

constipation, 81–82, 180

convulsions, 180

copper, colloidal, 137

coronary heart dis-ease, 180

cortisol, 26, 97

coughing, 180

cramps, 68

crisis measures, in modern medicine, 46–47

Cymatics, 49

dairy products, 36, 90, 96, 119

dancing, 148

"dead" foods, 37, 59, 65, 69, 70, 125

deficiencies

    light, 17, 26, 27–28. *See also* I.D. Therapy (Interactive Determination Therapy)

    mineral, 24

degenerative/destructive patterns, 135–136

dental problems, 180

depression, 180

detoxification process

    healing symptoms in, 67–70, 80–81

    pharmaceuticals in, 68, 83

    toxins leaving body in, 68–69, 79–83

diabetes, 4, 180

diarrhea, 68, 180

diets, 59, 118

digestible nutrients, 81

digestive system, 87–94

    digestive process and, 88–92

    dis-ease conditions in, 4, 56–57, 80, 86

    problems of, 92

    in Raphaology, 4

    repairing herbs/boosting foods, 93–94, 123

    role of, 87–88

    storage problem in, 4, 80, 86–87, 90–92

    stress and, 91, 92, 145

dis-ease

    accountability for, 9–10, 54, 55, 69–70, 72, 74, 103, 142

    decision to heal, 151–154

    in digestive system, 4, 56–57, 80, 86

    foods in overcoming, 56–57

    nutrients in healing, 65–66

    predispositions, 135, 136

    as preventable, 2

    as product of toxicity, 80

    symptoms of, 86, 90–91

Disney, Walt, 26
diverticulitis, 82
dizziness, 180
DNA (deoxyribonucleic acid), 133–139
Dolley, Stephen, Jr., 5
dormant immune factors, 135–136
dreams, 150
drug addiction/alcoholism, 178
dry skin, 180
duodenum, 89, 91

ear infection, 180
ectopic pregnancy, 128–129
eczema, 181
Edison, Thomas E., 11
ejaculation, 132
electrolytes, 97, 107, 110, 124
electromagnetic spectrum, 22–24, 26, 27, 30–31
electrons (enzymes), 24
e-motions (energy motions), 101–103
    heart and, 7
    light energy and, 17, 27–28, 141, 143
    positive versus harmful, 59
Emoto, Masaru, 20
endocrine glands, 16–17, 94–99
endometrium, 128–129
endorphins, 148
energetic intuitive powers, 6–7
energy increase, 181
Environmental Health and Light Research Institute, 26
enzymes, 22, 24, 31, 32–33, 35
    communication system and, 103
    in digestible nutrients, 81, 89
    in digestive process, 88–89, 92
    high enzyme foods, 83, 146–147, 166–169
    Peak Frequency Plant Therapy and, 33

gonadotropins, 96

gonads, 127

gonorrhea, 181

gout, 181

grave poaching, as basis of medical research, 45–46

green light, thyroid gland and, 17, 96

growth hormones, 95

hair, 120, 122–123

    health of, 122

    layers of, 122

    liver and, 120, 122

    role of, 122

hangover, 181

headache, 181

    in healing process, 69, 80, 81

healing symptoms, 67–70

    accountability for health conditions, 69–70

    detoxification process and, 67–69, 80–81

    role of, 67–68

    toxic stimulants and, 69

    toxins leaving body, 68–69, 79–83

    types of, 67–69, 72

health, definition of, 15, 152

heart

    in Body Banter, 76

    brain and, 7, 76

    chambers of, 113

    in circulatory system, 112–113

    in communication system, 100, 101

    e-motions (energy motions) and, 7

    nervous system and, 100, 101

    repairing herbs/boosting foods, 104, 114, 171

    respiration and, 109–110

    role of, 7, 76, 112–113

heartbeat rate, 97, 113

heartburn, 81, 181

heart problems, 66, 180, 181

hemoglobin, 109–110

hemorrhoids, 181

herbs

    antibacterial, 82

    defined, 33

    in detoxification process, 68, 83

    in extract/liquid form, 93–94, 108, 114, 120, 126

    fear of, 51–52

    nature of, 33–34

    powers of, 70, 82

    in Raphaology medicine, 3, 6, 11–12, 33–35, 147, 170–171

    role of, 34

    types of, 33–34

herpes/fever blister, 181

hippocampus, 101–102

hives, 181

Hollowich, Fritz, 26

Honey Mustard Dressing, 176–177

hormone system, 16–18, 94–99

    colors associated with specific glands, 16–17

    as fuel for organs, 17

    light energy and, 16–18, 22, 26–28, 30

    main hormone producing glands, 16–17, 94–99. *See also names of specific glands*

    nature of, 16, 94

    role of, 28, 85–86

    stress hormones, 26, 97, 125

hot flashes, 181

HRT (hormone replacement therapy), 182

Humane Genome Project, 134–135, 137–138

hunger, 72

hydrochloric acid, 89

hymen, 131

hypothalamus, 101–102

I.D. Therapy (Interactive Determination Therapy), 12, 37–38
idealization, 150
ileitis, 82
immune dis-ease, 182
immune system, 21, 33, 81, 104–108. *See also* pineal gland
    digestive system and, 91
    dormant factors, 135–136
    germ theory and, 58
    light energy and, 30
    repairing herbs/boosting foods, 108
immunoglobulin, 105
independence, importance of, 9–10
indigenous healing plants, as basis of Raphaology, 3, 6, 11–12
indigestible nutrients, 81
indigestion, 182
industrial waste, 33
infections, 53, 74, 82, 182
infertility, 182
infinite life source potential, 141–144
inflammation, 182
influenza, 182
inner ear, repairing herbs/boosting foods, 171
insect bite, 182
insomnia, 182
intuitive energetic powers
    nature of, 6
    in Raphaology, 6–7
involuntary functions, 73, 85
irregularity, 81–82
irritable bowels, 81–82, 182
Italian Anti-Acid Dressing, 176
Italian Blend, 173

Jenny, Hans, 48–49
Johnson, Milbank, 48
joint problems, 182

RAPHAOLOGY *Nature's Antidote for Commercialized Medicine*

APPENDIX B

The following chart is a copyright of Raphaology

How To Read the Chart:

The **<u>Color</u>** column represents the color of light in the spectrum of frequencies from which glands in the human body make their hormones.

The **<u>Gland/Organ</u>** column represents the specific systems consisting of hormone producing glands and their corresponding life support organs that use the spectrum of light in its field for healing.

The **<u>Herb</u>** column represents the single herb that contains the specific property for repairing the gland or organ directly in line across from the listed body part.

The **<u>Food</u>** column represents the one food that boosts the function of the corresponding body part directly across the line.

As light enters the physical body through the pituitary gland, the master hormone supervisor, and separates out into the spectrum of colors, each one passes down the matrix of light/hormone centers to furnish each gland and system organ with the energy to perform its peak function.

This differs even from the common practice of treating symptoms that originate from an organ by viewing health from a holistic perspective, taking into consideration that the hormone producing glands furnish hormones that fuel each organ function. This is important because if hormones are out of balance, the corresponding organs become dysfunctional. Treating organs alone without going to the causal gland/hormone is insufficient. Healing takes place with the all-encompassing combinations of herbs and foods.

RAPHAOLOGY Nature's Antidote for Commercialized Medicine

acceptance in germ theory, 58
spectrum frequencies in destroying, 47–48
vibration in destroying, 49
anti-clotting, 178
anti-depressant, 178
anti-histamine, 178
anxiety, 178
appendicitis, 178
appendix
repairing herbs/boosting foods, 93, 108, 171
role of, 105–106
apples, 36
arrhythmias, 178
art
defined, 39
healing arts, 41–43. *See also* Raphaology medicine
nature of, 39, 40
origins of, 40
West versus East and, 41
arteries
repairing herbs/boosting foods, 104
role of, 111
arteriosclerosis, 111
arthritis, 4, 123, 179
asthma, 4, 90–91, 179
atherosclerosis, 64–65
athlete's foot, 179
auric spectrum, 20–22, 30

back/muscle ache, 179
Back to Eden (Kloss), 52–53
bacteria
antibacterial herbs, 82
super resistant, 48
bad breath, 179
bananas, de-gassing, 107, 119

RAPHAOLOGY *Nature's Antidote for Commercialized Medicine*

quality of food and, 68–69
epididymis, 131–132
erythroprotein, 125
estrogen, 98, 128
exercise, 110, 116, 131, 148
eyes, repairing herbs/boosting foods, 93, 171

fallopian tubes, 128–130
fantasies, 150
Fat-Burner Dressing, 176
fats, 22
    quality of, 118
    role of, 118
fatty acids
    in digestive process, 88–90, 92
    sources of, 161
fear, 181
fertilization process, 128–129
fever, 181
    in healing process, 68, 80, 107
fever blisters, 181
fiber, in digestive process, 92
fimbriae, 130
fluoridated water, 24, 33
follicle stimulating hormones (FSH), 128
Food and Drug Administration (FDA), 51, 52, 64
food poisoning, 68
foods
    absence in modern medicine, 47
    "dead," 37, 59, 65, 69, 70, 125
    defined, 33
    fake, 86–87
    fatty acid sources, 161
    foods to avoid, 159–160
    genetically modified (GMO), 33, 36–37
    marketing of, 36–37

gonadotropins, 96
gonads, 127
gonorrhea, 181
gout, 181
grave poaching, as basis of medical research, 45–46
green light, thyroid gland and, 17, 96
growth hormones, 95

hair, 120, 122–123
    health of, 122
    layers of, 122
    liver and, 120, 122
    role of, 122
hangover, 181
headache, 181
    in healing process, 69, 80, 81
healing symptoms, 67–70
    accountability for health conditions, 69–70
    detoxification process and, 67–69, 80–81
    role of, 67–68
    toxic stimulants and, 69
    toxins leaving body, 68–69, 79–83
    types of, 67–69, 72
health, definition of, 15, 152
heart
    in Body Banter, 76
    brain and, 7, 76
    chambers of, 113
    in circulatory system, 112–113
    in communication system, 100, 101
    e-motions (energy motions) and, 7
    nervous system and, 100, 101
    repairing herbs/boosting foods, 104, 114, 171
    respiration and, 109–110
    role of, 7, 76, 112–113
heartbeat rate, 97, 113

RAPHAOLOGY *Nature's Antidote for Commercialized Medicine*

joints

      repairing herbs/boosting foods, 119, 182

      role of, 116–117

Keightly, Alan, 141

Ketchup, Raw, 175–176

kidney dis-ease, 117–118, 123, 182

kidney infection, 182

kidneys

      in detoxification process, 80

      location of, 17, 94, 97

      repairing/boosting herb formulas, 99

      repairing herbs/boosting foods, 97, 108, 123, 126, 171

      role of, 92

      skin and, 120, 124

      stress hormones and, 26, 97, 125

      in urinary system, 124

      violet light and, 17, 97

kidney stones, 117–118, 182

killer immune cells, 96, 104–105, 107

kitchen

      adding items to, 157–159

      removing items from, 156–157

Klenner, Fred R., 66

Kloss, Jethro, 52–53

knowledge, as power, 10

labia, 130–131

laboratory tests, 38, 77

Lao Tzu, 71

laughter, 147

leukocytes, 104–105

ligaments, 116

ligand, 102

light energy

      auric spectrum and, 20–22, 30

as basis of Raphaology medicine, 11–12, 13, 29–38, 49–50. *See also* Color Therapy

cells and, 18, 20, 30, 49–50

colors and. *See* colors; Color Therapy

cycle of light in human body, 21

deficiencies of, 17, 26, 27–28

defined, 29

distortion of, 24, 26, 29–31

e-motions and, 17, 27–28, 141, 143

hormones and, 16–18, 22, 26–28, 30

importance of, 29–30

mineral light, 22–24, 31

physics of light, 19–24

prismatic fluid and, 20–22, 27

sunlight, 21–22, 24, 29, 31

symptoms of adequate, 17, 27–28

symptoms of deficiencies, 17, 27–28

types of, 29. *See also* sunlight

light spectrum, 31

limbic system, 101

Lipton, Bruce, 135, 137–138

liver

digestible nutrients and, 81

hair and, 120, 122

repairing herbs/boosting foods, 93, 123, 171

role of, 89–90, 92

stress hormones and, 26

liver dis-ease, 90, 182

living matter

defined, 50

as vibrating form, 50–54

love

importance of, 149–150

self-love, 149

lungs

in detoxification process, 80

in immune system, 106
    repairing herbs/boosting foods, 108, 114, 123, 171
    role of, 106, 109–110, 111, 112
lymphatic function, 96–97, 111, 112
    repairing herbs/boosting foods, 114, 171
lymph nodes, 104
    repairing herbs/boosting foods, 108
    role of, 106–107
lymphocytes, 104–105

macrophages, 104–105
magnetic fields, 22, 141
malnutrition, 26, 33, 81
    deficiency symptoms, 65
    defined, 4
    drug treatment for, 66
mammary glands, 96–97
    blue light and, 17, 97
    location of, 17, 94, 96–97
    repairing/boosting herb formulas, 99, 110, 171
    repairing herbs/boosting foods, 97
Marden, Orlson Swett, 55
master gland. *See* pituitary gland
Mayonnaise, 175
medicine. *See* modern medicine; Raphaology medicine
meditation, 66
melanin, 95
melatonin, 26–27, 96
memory, 73, 101, 102
memory loss, 182
menopause, 98, 183
menstruation, 129–130, 183
metabolism, 89, 96
metastasis, 52
Mexican Blend, 173
migraines, 183

muscles
>repairing herbs/boosting foods, 120
>role of, 115–116
music, 147–148

nail problems, 123–124, 183
nails, 120, 123–124
>repairing herbs/boosting foods, 123–124
Napoleon Bonaparte, 45
nature, 148–149
nausea, 183
>in healing process, 68, 81
nephrons, 124
nervousness, 183
nervous system
>repairing herbs/boosting foods, 104
>role of, 100
neti pot therapy, 107
neuropeptides, 101–103
neurotransmitters, 103
nipples. *See* mammary glands
nutrients
>categories of, 22
>digestible, 81
>impact in healing dis-ease, 65–66
>indigestible, 81

obesity, 90, 183
olfactory, repairing herbs/boosting foods, 171
orange light, pancreas and, 17, 98
organs. *See also names of specific organs*
>in Body Banter, 74, 75–78
>in detoxification process, 80
>herbs and, 34–35
>hormones and, 85–86
>hormones as fuel for, 17

introducing brain to, 72–74
light energy and, 17
Raphaology Chart, 170–171
stress and, 82
toxins trapped in, 80
Ornish, Dean, 66
Osler, William, 61
osteoarthritis, 183
osteoporosis, 4
Ott, John N., 26
ovaries. *See* testes and ovaries
overdoses, 65
oviducts, 128–129
ovulation, 128, 130, 131
ovum, 127, 131
oxygen, 109–110

pain, 53, 183
    in healing process, 69
    role of, 74
pancreas
    in digestive process, 89, 91–92
    location of, 17, 94, 97
    orange light and, 17, 98
    repairing/boosting herb formulas, 99
    repairing herbs/boosting foods, 93, 108, 171
    role of, 89, 91–92, 97–98, 106, 108
pancreas dis-ease, 4, 91, 183
pancreas duct, repairing herbs/boosting foods, 171
pancreatitis, 4
parasites, 104
parathyroid gland, 96
Pauling, Linus, 66
Peak Frequency Foods, 35–36, 68–69, 146–147
    list of, 166–169
    21 day peak frequency food challenge, 163–165

INDEX

repairing herbs/boosting foods, 110, 171
role of, 109–110
Rife, Royal Raymond, 47–48
Rife Ray Machine, 48
RNA (ribonucleic acid), 137
runny nose, in healing process, 80

salad dressings, 176–177
Fat Burner Dressing, 176
French Fat Burner Dressing, 177
Honey Mustard Dressing, 176–177
Italian Anti-Acid Dressing, 176
saliva, 88
salivary enzymes, 88
salt, 24, 96, 100, 125–126. *See also* Real Salt™
Schweitzer, Albert, 85
science. *See also* modern medicine
defined, 39
impact of, 40–41
nature of, 39, 40
origins of, 39–40
West versus East and, 41
scrotum, 127, 131
scurvy, 64–65
Seafood Blend, 172–173
sebeceous glands, 121
self-love, 149
semen, 132
seminal fluid, 132
sensory information, 101
serotonin, 95
sex glands. *See* testes and ovaries
sex organs. *See* testes and ovaries
sinews, 116
sinuses
repairing herbs/boosting foods, 171

INDEX

spontaneous remissions/recoveries, 42–43

Stanford University, 138

Stanley, Edward, 67

STD (sexually transmitted disease), 184

stem cells, 127, 128

steroid production, 26

stimulants, 69

stomach

      repairing herbs/boosting foods, 93, 171

      role of, 106

stomach problems, 184

stool softener, 184

stress, 64–65, 66, 70, 145–150, 184

      adrenals and, 26, 97, 125

      B-Complex Vitamins, 82, 98

      causes of, 145–146

      communication system and, 102, 103

      digestive system and, 91, 92, 145

      impact of, 82

      indigestible nutrients and, 81–82

      methods of reducing, 146–150

      pancreas and, 98

      reducing, 83

stress hormones, 26, 97, 125

structural system, 115–120

      bones in, 115, 116–120

      joints in, 116–117, 119, 182

      ligaments in, 116

      muscles in, 115–116, 120

      repairing herbs/boosting foods, 119–120

stuffy nose, in healing process, 80, 107

sugars. *See* carbohydrates

sunlight

      as energy source, 21–22, 24, 29, 31

      plants and, 22

sunscreens, 31, 118

Tomlin, Lily, 145

tonsils
  repairing herbs/boosting foods, 93, 108, 171
  role of, 88, 106, 107

toothache/abscess, 184

touch, 121, 147

toxicity theory, 57–59

toxic shock, 184

toxins. *See also* immune system
  circulatory system and, 111
  detoxification process and, 67–69, 79–83
  digestive storage problem and, 4, 80, 86–87, 90–92
  process of leaving body, 68–69, 79–83
  reproductive organs and, 98, 99

tryptophan, 95

tubiligation, 128–129

tumor arrest, 184

21 day peak frequency food challenge, 163–165

ulcers, 81, 184

ultra-violet light, 22, 26, 118

University of Southern California (USC), 48

ureters
  repairing herbs/boosting foods, 126
  in urinary system, 124

urethra, 124, 131–133

uric acid, 124

urinary system, 124–126
  components of, 124–126. *See also* adrenals; bladder;
kidneys; ureters
  role of, 124

urinary tract infection, 184

urine, 125

uterus, 98, 128–130

vaccines, 33

RAPHAOLOGY *Nature's Antidote for Commercialized Medicine*

energies in, 20
high-frequency words and, 20, 21
quality of, 20–21, 78
in respiration, 110
in skin hydration, 121–122
urinary system and, 125
White, E. B., 9
white blood cells
repairing herbs/boosting foods, 171
role of, 104–108
white light, 20, 27
whooping cough, 185
Wilczek, Frank, 19
Wolf, Jonathan: Thunder, 12–13, 47, 49–50, 74
words, high-frequency, 20, 21, 50
World Health Organization (WHO), 15
wounds, 185
wrinkles, 185

X-rays, 38

yeast infection, 185
yellow light, pineal gland and, 16, 96

Zeis optics, 47
Zeno, 29